AF225249

Death By
Chocolate Cake

MY JOURNEY THROUGH OBESITY WITH LOVE

Jenny Marshall

All rights reserved. No part of this book may be used or reproduced, stored in a retrieval system, or transmitted in any form or by any means, electronic, mechanical, photocopying, recording, scanning, or otherwise, without written permission from the publisher except in the case of brief quotations embodied in critical articles and reviews. Permission for wider usage of this material can be obtained through Quoir by emailing permission@quoir.com.

Copyright © 2021 by Jenny Marshall.

First Edition

Cover design and layout by Rafael Polendo (polendo.net)

All names have been changed for legal reasons and to protect the privacy of those individuals.

All Scripture quotations, unless otherwise indicated, are taken from the *Holy Bible, New International Version*®, NIV®. Copyright ©1973, 1978, 1984, 2011 by Biblica, Inc.™ Used by permission of Zondervan. All rights reserved worldwide. www.zondervan.comThe "NIV" and "New International Version" are trademarks registered in the United States Patent and Trademark Office by Biblica, Inc.™

ISBN 978-1-938480-84-3

This volume is printed on acid free paper and meets ANSI Z39.48 standards.

Printed in the United States of America

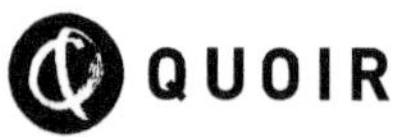

Published by Quoir
Oak Glen, California

www.quoir.com

Dedication

Dedicated to Althea, Diana, Jeff and Willie who offered their love and support through the most difficult times.

And to my parents who I love deeply and survived their own trauma.

Table of Contents

Foreword

I have devoted the last thirty years of my life counseling, coaching, mentoring, guiding, and teaching people all over the world in the area of personal growth and development, and have never encountered anyone who has experienced the degree of transformation and liberation than Jenny Marshall. Her life journey is so extraordinary and profound that I challenged her to tell her story. This book is that story.

Despite the abuse and severe maltreatment of her childhood and youth, despite the rejection, bullying, and persecution from grade-school to college, despite the contempt, derision, and discrimination she endured in the workforce, Jenny ultimately prevailed.

What was her "sin"?

Obesity.

From an early age, Jenny found refuge in food from a family of verbal, emotional, and mental abuse and as a comfort for the sexual abuse she endured. By the age of 12 she weighed 300 pounds, and reached 600 pounds as an adult. Her obesity was life-threatening. Turning to God in desperation, she joined a church only to endure more judgement, condemnation, and shame. Jenny was told that her obesity was a "sin"—a spiritual problem that could only be rectified through greater devotion to God. Despite all her religious effort, when no significant progress was made, Jenny was told she was afflicted by demons, and was traumatically subjected to an exorcism that was performed on her.

Jenny tried everything she knew and was told to do, including seeking God, but her food addiction persisted and she continued putting on weight. Her life was in jeopardy but Jenny had run out of reasons for wanting to live.

You wouldn't know any of this about Jenny if you met her today. She is a physically and mentally healthy person, earned undergraduate and graduate degrees, is a Finance and Human Resources manager, and runs her own accounting business on the side. She is also an adjunct college math and accounting instructor, and does individual counseling and coaching with people who suffer the physical and psychological effects of obesity.

So what happened?

What turned Jenny's life around? How does one explain the remarkable metamorphosis of her life? That's the story Jenny shares in this book.

I first met Jenny online, when she joined a cohort group I was leading on the subject of authentic self-expression. During that cohort experience I challenged her to consider writing about her life. I could clearly see that Jenny's astounding personal transformation was a remarkable human interest story that would inspire and help others. Jenny told me she was an accountant and not a writer, but she gave writing a chance and discovered she had a knack for it. I encouraged and supported Jenny through the process of putting her story to words, which wasn't an easy task as it opened several wounds and traumatic memories from her past. But she persisted with the project, which resulted in the book you are now holding, *Death by Chocolate Cake*.

Jenny has had a profound impact on my own life. Countless times along the way she explained to me that her greatest liberation was not losing weight and the transformation of her body, but losing shame and the transformation of her heart. Before and After pictures only depict the radical physical changes she underwent, not the whole, healthy, free, loving, wise, compassionate, and caring person she became inside.

Through Jenny I learned that virtually everything I thought I knew about obesity was wrong. There are countless misconceptions about the factors and dynamics that contribute to obesity. The idea that obesity is primarily the result of lack of self-discipline, gluttony, or other character flaws is grossly misinformed, and fails to grasp all the pivotal genetic and environmental variables that contribute to obesity, as well as the dynamics and cycle of addiction. Jenny also helped me understand the emotional and psychological factors at the root of obesity. It would not be an exaggeration to say that Jenny Marshall has an unparalleled and comprehensive knowledge of obesity, forged in the crucible of her personal experience and her in-depth involvement in the scientific, medical, physical, and mental health fields and communities.

Despite all that, what I most appreciate about Jenny is her sense of humor, accepting and loving disposition, genuine and deep spirituality, and her gentle and empathetic spirit.

The subtitle of *Death by Chocolate Cake* is *My Journey Through Obesity with Love*. At first I didn't care for this subtitle. I thought it needed more flash and pop. Eventually, I got it. Jenny attributes her unprecedented rebirth to love. If that doesn't sound too monumental it may be that you don't really understand love, at least not in the way Jenny discovered it.

Gary Zukav wrote, "Eventually you will come to understand that love heals everything, and love is all there is." I don't think I would have ever truly discovered this without Jenny. My hope is that in reading this book you will discover it too.

– **Jim Palmer**

Prologue

What Is Love?

Is love a feeling? Is it a being? Is it a knowing? For me, love is a being which comes from my innermost part, invading, pervading and pursuing me. It melds its way through those parts of me which I consider my darkest, discovering my hidden places and changing me deeply. Love is what I need it to be.

It forges its way into my heart, changing the thoughts which prevent its entrance into the deepest part of my soul. It is beautiful, exquisite, simple, pure, in me, of me, an integral part of me, yet not like me.

It knows me, understands me, cares for me, empathises with me and embraces me. It is always there, even when I am unaware of it. It never leaves me despite how I feel or what I am doing. Nothing can thwart its purpose. It will continue drawing me until I give in to its innate beauty. It is persistent and patient, kind and knowing. It is everything good, yet accepting of my guilt, fear and shame.

It is the strong sense of well-being, the warm feeling of belonging within me. It feels as if it belongs in me, I belong in it and I belong in myself. It forges my self-acceptance, keeping me from the war within myself. It understands what I do not know about myself. It keeps me from self-harm and abuse, withholding my weapons of personal warfare.

Given a chance, it consumes me, devouring my negativity and engaging me in a deep intimacy so personal that I feel captured in the moment.

This is love to me.

– Jenny Marshall

Introduction

Breaking My Silence

This is my story of how love changed my life. The world is filled with love stories, and what might first come to mind is a romance filled with passion. My journey is a love story, because it was love that gave me my life.

Writing my story was difficult, at times agonizing. I was an unhappy child and youth; this misery extended into my adulthood. Although writing this book meant reliving that nightmare, I decided to break my silence about my life's journey. Love had the last word, and I felt that deserved to be shared.

My addiction to food began as a child. In a dysfunctional family, I discovered that eating afforded me an escape from my reality. It offered relief, comfort, and good feelings. By the time I had reached 12 years of age, I weighed 300 pounds (132 kg). This made me an object of bullying and rejection at school, and I hated myself.

Life was a vicious cycle. I would drown my hurt and self-hatred with food, which made me feel good for the moment. This was followed by self-condemning guilt and shame self-talk, which created more tormenting feelings requiring more food. Eventually, I ate my way to morbid obesity.

By the time I reached adulthood my self-confidence had been destroyed by my weight. My physical and mental health suffered, my social life was non-existent, career opportunities were thwarted, and my faith was questioned because of my failure to overcome my addiction to food. We live in a world that is cruel to people who are grossly overweight. We judge them, ridicule them, scorn them, and exclude them. This was my world.

We all know the saying, "A journey of a thousand miles begins with a single step." The process of changing my life began with a few short steps, tentative at first. I am often asked the "secret" behind losing so much weight. It was not dieting, or a fitness program or medical intervention. The process required a new relationship with my body, with food and exercise.

The "secret" behind the transformation of my life was realizing that the root cause of my obesity was shame, and this prevented me from accepting love. Obesity was who I was and what I was supposed to be. It was familiar and afforded me security. My obesity kept people at a distance, which was okay by me. I had stopped believing that I belonged and was not going to risk rejection again.

In Australia where I live, 67 percent of adults are overweight or obese. Over 25 percent of children and adolescents aged 2-17 are overweight or obese. The health risks associated with obesity are many; they include an increased risk of death from all causes, hypertension, type 2 diabetes, heart disease, stroke, osteoarthritis, and several types of cancer. Together, obesity and being overweight is the second leading cause of preventable death in Australia.

There was an assortment of contributing factors that led to my weight gain, including genetics and psychological trauma. But what kept me from addressing it was shame.

Shame is the intensely painful feeling from believing that we are flawed and therefore unworthy of love. It is caused by toxic beliefs about us that are deeply connected to our sense of who we are. Shame says I am ... defective, unlovable, worthless, no-good, a failure, ugly, hopeless.

The pain of my childhood and adolescence drove me to eat. My dominating and angry dad, and my mum's untreated depression, overshadowed my early life. In the absence of security and love at home, food became my safe and happy place.

The more I ate and the heavier I became, the more my parents and siblings were ashamed of my size and weight, just as I was. Dad was merciless with his criticism and degrading names, shaming me for being overweight. Classmates at school mocked and bullied me. It was clear at the earliest age that I was ugly and someone to be despised. So, I ate.

I ate until food became an addiction. The portions of food I consumed grew larger, and the frequency of my eating increased. I ate even when I was no longer hungry. I would eat to the point of feeling ill. Sneaking food out of the kitchen and hiding my eating was a daily stress. I lived in constant anxiety about when I would eat again, and if the foods I craved would be available. I couldn't stop. The more I ate, the more obese I became, the more rejection I received, the more I hated myself … the more I ate.

Shaming from others did not work, every attempt to curb my eating and diet failed, the threat of serious illness and death did not stop me, even church did not help. I believed I was worthless and unlovable, so I lacked the motivation to help myself. After all, if I died, I thought no one could care.

Simply stated, my life was heading toward an early end.

Although the easiest part to see of my transformation was the weight loss, something much more profound happened within me. I discovered who I was through inner change and found a beautiful life within.

Chapter One
All You Need is Cake

The kitchen was filled with the aroma of freshly baked chocolate cake. As I turned it out onto the plate, the smell intensified. Impatient with desire, I iced it while it was still warm. The rich, thick chocolate frosting dripped down the sides and soaked into the cake, melting into it as it touched the warm surface. This was going to be beautiful. My mouth watered in expectation.

When it had cooled just enough, I carefully slid my knife into the cake. The thick slice came away with ease. It was just right—moist, dense, and soft with the icing melted into the centre.

The rich chocolate flavour wafted from the spoon to my nose. As soon as the cake touched my tongue, the flavour hit me. The soft texture was comforting. The warmth reminded me of mum's love. I missed her love, and I felt close to her as I ate. Eating made me feel connected with her and a part of myself which I had lost when she died.

My mind was transported back to my childhood. Mum was cooking, and I felt loved by her. She enjoyed cooking; it was her way of showing affection. Tenderness was not a thing in my family; mum's food became a substitute for it. Over time it came to represent many things to me. In fact, it became the solution to almost everything.

Then came the rush from the intensely sweet icing and I was brought back to the present moment. Feelings of euphoria came over me as I devoured the slice. I wasn't sure which I enjoyed the most—the euphoria from the sugar, or the nurture from eating food like mum once made. Either way, it was wonderful.

Before I'd finished the first, the second slice was already on my mind. There was no time to linger in the experience. I was on a high from sugar, my addiction had kicked in and I could not wait. I wanted more, now!

In that moment my pain was gone; I was anaesthetised. The thoughts which had haunted me all day were forgotten. I had been desperate for comfort, and now my desire was being satisfied.

Devouring the second slice, the flavour did not matter to me. My thoughts were focussed on the sugary rush, and I needed all the love and comfort I could get.

"Just one more piece", I thought, just as mum would say as she fought with her addiction demons. "No one is around, you can do this without anyone knowing," my thoughts continued.

But there would never be an end to this. There was not enough chocolate cake in the world to satisfy my need for love, and I could not quench my desire for sugar. The mixture of sugar and fat was a deadly substitute for love. It awakened an untamed part of me which I could not control.

In the middle of my third slice, I noticed the small voice of guilt howling in the distance. As I continued to eat, it became louder as if closer to me. But I kept eating. Then It was so loud that it almost smothered the comfort and euphoria.

As I struggled to hold myself back from another piece, I noticed only half was left. I had been intoxicated by the experience and blinded to what I was doing. The rich, moist, soft cake had lost its lustre, the expectation was gone, and guilt had taken its place. My emotions were a mixture of an unsatisfied desire for love, and shame for what I had done.

Punishing myself, the toxic shame took over, "You shouldn't do this. If you keep going you will get diabetes. You are fat and bad! You deserve all the mocking you have received. You should be ashamed of yourself…"

The cycle had completed itself. My chest was knotted with fear. I was alone, and no one loved me now.

From as early as I can remember, food had been my source of comfort. By my early teens it had developed into a full-blown addiction. I had an insatiable desire to eat, which controlled my life. Not only was I now seeking comfort, but I was addicted to the rush from sugar. I had reached a point where I was unable to recognise the 'hungry' or 'full' sensations in my stomach. I was a master at overeating, consuming large amounts at a time. Eating fast helped me elude attention, and savouring the flavour was not possible.

As a child I would lie to my parents about how much I had eaten. An expert at stealing food behind their back, I would hide chocolate or cookies in my bedroom after sneaking it from cupboards and countertops.

My feelings for food swung like a pendulum, starting with love, comfort and anaesthetising my pain. Then swinging to fear, shame, and self-punishment, sabotaging my life by deceiving me about myself.

This one piece of chocolate cake sums up my unhealthy relationship with food. But it was not the problem, it was the symptom. Like every addiction, it was a poor substitute for my need.

What did this piece of chocolate cake mean to me? It did not judge me, nor did it lecture me. It silently listened to me, nurturing me in the process. It understood my need and went some way to satisfying it.

Food was my substitute for love. Even though it never satisfied me, I used it constantly to fill the void within me. Addiction is like that;

it is not logical. This is what I have worked through on my journey out of shame.

The following chapters tell my story out of obesity and food addiction. Even if obesity is not something you struggle with, my journey may resonate with you. We all have something in our lives which seems too big to overcome. I hope you will find inspiration for whatever your battle is in life.

My desire is that this book will encourage you to face your own misplaced dependencies. I hope you are moved to work through your wounds and find healing and wholeness in your life. What I have to offer is understanding, acceptance, and love.

We all have our crude methods for managing our inner demons. Removing these things from our lives can only occur when they are faced head-on. It's a frightening proposition to face our demons. Healing takes courage, and we all have courage, even if we have to dig a little to find it.

What is your piece of chocolate cake? More importantly, what is your pain?

Chapter Two

Ghosts of Christmas Past

There are painful memories that time does not erase. The years do not make them forgettable, only bearable.

Thirty years on from my childhood, it was the week before Christmas, and I was finishing up the month-end financial reports where I worked. When I walked out the door that evening, I had two weeks of holidays ahead of me.

Despite the high temperatures in Australia, celebrations were beginning—Christmas lights and decorations adorned houses, stores were packed with last-minute shoppers, and families were making their holiday plans. Needing a few items from the supermarket, I pulled into a space near the front. As I got out of my car, I noticed a mother and her little girl walking through the car park. The mother was agitated and impatiently pulling her daughter along, cursing her under her breath.

Suddenly, memories of my childhood invaded my mind. I was transported back in time as a young girl. One particular Christmas day has especially haunted me over the years.

I was awake early on that Christmas morning, excited and eager to discover what was under the tree. "Can I open my presents mum?", I asked from my parents' bedroom door. "Yes, as long as you are quiet", mum called out in a frustrated tone. I heard nothing from dad's side of the room.

Mum had surrounded the Christmas tree with presents the night before, after I had gone to bed, each one wrapped in festive holiday wrapping paper. Red, green, and gold packages covered the floor. I found my pile of gifts and began unwrapping as mum watched on. Thrill and delight filled me as I discovered what was inside each package. "It's a Barbie Doll!", I yelped in joy as I opened the box to feel the long blonde hair, and marvel at her beautiful clothes.

When dad and brother were stirring, mum started breakfast. The smell of fried bacon and eggs, and toasting bread wafted through the house. She sat with them for Christmas breakfast, and when they had finished, mum cleared the table and washed the dishes. She also filled a platter with all kinds of yummy Christmas treats—potato crisps, nuts, candies, and chocolates.

As the house heated up, she switched on the air-conditioner to cool off the kitchen, which was roasting from the heat outside. There was no relief in sight, mum needed to start making a hot lunch. I watched as she busied herself preparing the meal with all the trimmings. She had made the brandy custard sauce and Christmas pudding the night before, so that lunch would be served at 12 pm sharp.

By late morning, the kitchen was filled with the aroma of roast chicken and pork. Vegetables were in the oven, and gravy was made from the meat juices bubbling on the stove. Mum sliced ham and buttered bread rolls. My sisters came to help. We all gathered around the table as a family to eat at 12 pm.

This may sound like a happy Christmas occasion, but you could cut the tension with a knife. One wrong move or untimely word could trigger an eruption of anger from either of my parents, and most likely end in an argument between them. Christmas was always when our family dysfunction was at its peak.

Before we sat down for lunch, I had already eaten the entire platter of Christmas goodies. Mum re-filled it. I re-ate it. My stomach was full by the time the meal was served. This was how I coped with the stress I carried inside.

Mum was seething with resentment, intermittently heaving it upon anyone who came near her. Her face was red with anger. She unleashed her fury about all she had to do. Whenever I asked if I could help, she complained that I was in the way.

An army of flies were buzzing around the outside screen door to the kitchen, awaiting their opportunity to get into the food. When my brother came through the screen door, the expectant flies took the opportunity. Mum was fuming and threw a curse at my brother.

Meanwhile, dad was sulking. He was infuriated about all the money spent over Christmas. He angrily raved on about how expensive and pointless it was, and a waste of time when he could be working to make more money. He criticised mum for the cost of Christmas, accused us of expecting too much, and swore at me for overeating.

On the last Christmas we shared as a family, mum worked slavishly to get the food on the table by noon. To irritate her, dad decided to drive around the farm, taking my brother and one of my sisters with him. They eventually came inside, about an hour late for lunch. Mum was furious, and deeply hurt.

Mum, my other sister, and I ate lunch together in silence. Dad eventually came in, along with the others, and ate his lunch in the usual arrogant way. We listened to his commentary about how moody mum was, and how we were to blame because we didn't help her. I didn't utter a word, I believed it was my fault. I disappeared inside myself and I shovelled more of the rich food down.

Sitting in my car outside the supermarket, I watched the indignant mother pulling her daughter through the sliding front door. Feelings of sadness slowly washed through me like cold rain.

I learned as a little girl that it was not okay to express what I felt. My most tender emotions were met with mum's indifference and dad's anger. Vulnerability was demeaned. I didn't have the right to feel anything but guilt and shame. I could not show or voice my feelings, so I ate instead.

The guilt and shame came with me when I left home. The weight of mum's unhappiness was unbearable. When she died, I felt responsible. I blamed myself for her misery. Perhaps if I had been a better daughter, she would have been happier and even lived longer.

Grieving the ghosts of Christmases past has not come easily. Grief is always messy. One emotion doesn't flow neatly into another; it hits suddenly. The pain comes in never ending waves and the only way to make it stop is to feel it deeply.

My childhood broke my heart, but I eventually learned it was not broken like shattered pieces; it was broken open like an oyster shell to reveal a priceless treasure inside. It's a treasure that you have too.

Chapter Three
Fear of Dad

He stood in the darkened doorway, pointing his cigarette at me like a weapon. The smell of the smoke drifted towards my bed, and the glowing ashes fell to the floor as he shook it at me. "You bitch!", he said, "You've upset your mother now and she's sick. If you ever do that again, I'll break your bloody neck!"

This was dad's reaction to an incident earlier in the evening, when I stood on top of the ottoman when my cousin was visiting. "Get off that, you bloody big fat lump!", he had yelled, embarrassed that my morbid obesity was on display to his relatives.

I was 16 at the time. I should have known better. This was not the first-time dad had erupted like this. After his explosion, I burst into tears and rushed to my bedroom, meeting mum along the way. "What's happened?" she'd asked angrily. "Dad just called me a bloody big fat lump", I said sobbing. Mum was furious.

Lying in bed, my gut was tied in knots of guilt and fear. A while later, I heard the floor creaking in the hallway leading to my room. I wondered if dad had come to apologize. Instead, this is when he unleashed his verbal attack at my bedroom door.

Dad hated me. He never told me that he loved me. He always found something about me to criticise, especially my weight. To dad, I was slow, fat, and the reason for his and mum's misery. But instead of being angry with dad, I was angry with myself. If I had not been overweight, none of this would have happened. It was my fault.

Dad was a callous man. He grew up in a farming family that lived in an arid region of Australia. His parents had worked the land when the area was sparsely populated and considered remote. He helped his father clear the land by dragging chains between two horses to knock down trees. With hot, dry and barren conditions, it made farming strenuous and unforgiving.

He resented his father who he said had made his life on the farm tortuous, and finances tight for mum and himself. His dad was a harsh, demanding and critical man. Many years removed; I was able to see that dad treated me in the same way he was dealt with. Wounded people, wound others.

Mum and dad's relationship was turbulent. Mum had carried her own wounds into their relationship. They were going through a traumatic time before my birth, which shook their marriage. Mum had a miscarriage, and they were on the verge of losing the family farm, which brought out the worst in them.

Losing the farm would have meant the loss of the only world dad had ever known. More and more debt was accumulating, but he managed to save most of the farm by selling off a strip of land to a neighbouring farmer. He learned a new trade, and eventually paid off the debt and built a small empire. Dad worked incessantly, claiming it was necessary. But he kept long hours and worked weekends to avoid mum and facing the problems of their marriage. He became obsessed with his empire and money.

My parents met through dad's mother. While visiting the city to visit her brother, she crossed paths with mum and struck up a conversation. In a manner typical of her country background she invited mum to stay on the farm. Dad was sent to pick her up at the train station. Mum admired dad's strength; he could lift two bags of wheat on his shoulders at one time. One evening mum could not undo the taps to fill the bathtub. Dad's mother told him to help. As the story goes, that's when they fell in love, in the bathroom, over the tub.

Their marriage date was set, but dad did not attend any wedding rehearsals. The ceremony was scheduled in February, which was the reaping season. The minister asked mum if dad was going to be there on the day of the wedding. He came, with a white forehead from wearing a hat during harvest, and a body that was dark tan.

Every few years my dad would buy a new high-end Ford. Yet, we lived in an old, dilapidated house which he did not update. At one point the house was so run-down that the walls in the bedrooms cracked at the joins, and bits of plaster came adrift. Bees swarmed in the vents, forcing us to wear shoes in the bedrooms, and check our beds before sleep to avoid being stung.

The toilet was an add-on. There were no windows, just two holes made by a gap in the bricks for ventilation. If the wind was in the right direction, rain would fall through the gaps, soaking our back as we sat. The sewerage pit, which was just outside the toilet window, would overflow sending effluent along a winding course beyond the lawn, over an access road and into the paddock beside the house. Not only did the best lawn grow along this course, but the juiciest tomatoes grew from seeds in the effluent at the end of the flow.

The laundry floor was poorly laid. Water from the twin-tub washing machine would sit in the centre of the floor rather than going down the drain. When mum was washing, she stood in the water and got shocks from the washing machine.

Dad was a bully. He was the kind of man who blamed others and was never wrong. Possessions were more important to him than his family. He could be ruthless and cruel verbally, mocking and ridiculing me for fun. We rarely had an interaction or conversation that didn't include him demeaning me. After all, I was the problem child in the family because I was the youngest female and the fattest. I avoided time alone with dad because I was afraid of him.

Deep down, there was nothing I wanted more than to please dad. As a young girl I desperately wanted to feel special to him, but instead I was shown disfavour and indifference. I perpetually fell short of his expectations, regardless of how hard I tried to earn his approval.

The fear of his rejection paralysed me. I walked a tightrope, trying to avoid upsetting him. To lose balance meant I would fall into the burning hell of dad's wrath. I learned to steer clear and hide from him.

When I turned 13, dad decided to have a "chat" with me. He took me for a drive, alone. As I sat beside him in the car my gut tightened with fear. Being alone with dad was terrifying. His rage and shame-filled comments frightened me. I braced myself for what was coming. While we were driving out toward an old water well, he talked to me about my "condition". He was referring to my weight.

"You've got too much condition on you", he said in a gruff voice. This is how dad talked about his horses. If they were in good condition, this meant they were healthy and had the ideal amount of fat on them. Having "too much condition" meant they were overweight and wouldn't perform well. He continued angrily, "That's what you are. You need to do something about it."

I sat quietly, slowly dying inside. Crying was not an option. After a few minutes, he continued, "I got to about 18 stone and I was too bloody big! I got sugar diabetes and did something about it before it killed me. You need to do the bloody same," he said in an irate voice. I nodded in acknowledgment, too afraid to utter a word.

He was ashamed of me. His words cut me to the core. To dad, I was nothing more than a fat worthless horse. His comments about diabetes and death made me afraid of dying. When we returned home, I retreated to my room.

There was no point hating dad; doing this would dig me deeper into the pain caused by our relationship. But, as painful as it was, honesty with myself and understanding him was the only path for me to healing. Looking back, I can see that he was a broken and empty man. He externalised his need for significance by pressuring his children to perform and shamed them if they failed. In those times, a man was partly judged by the character and attributes of his children. My obesity was a constant disgrace to him. I had dishonoured his public reputation.

I emerged from my childhood believing I was a failure. My obesity was not something I occasionally did that let dad down. My obesity was a "condition"—it was who I was every minute, of every hour, of every day. It wasn't that I did bad things, it was that who and what I was essentially was bad, shameful, and worthless. I could never be good enough to be loved.

Growing up with dad's condemnation poisoned my relationship with myself, men and God. I could not accept myself because my own father could not. My fear of failure plagued me at every turn.

My belief that I was unlovable and unworthy was firmly entrenched. It never occurred to me that my own father's genetics and struggles with food and weight, may have contributed to my obesity. Nor did I consider that the trauma of our relationship, and the dysfunction of the family could have been psychological factors that fuelled my food addiction.

My conclusion was that I was obese because I was bad. There wasn't anything that could be done. This is who I was. So, I just kept eating.

Chapter Four

Food Is Love

Every day at school was stressful. I had few friends, felt shunned by classmates, and frequently a target of ridicule and bullying. Humiliating names were hurled at me across the school yard. Teachers disregarded me. I spent lunch and recess breaks alone.

At the end of another difficult day, the school bus dropped me off at the top of our farm driveway. A dirt road lined with pine trees led to our house. Even though it was only a short walk, mum was in her usual spot waiting. She was relieved to see me after a day mostly on her own.

As I got into the car, she asked, "How was your day, Bubby?" I told her it was fine. This was my standard response. It was not safe to divulge my true feelings with mum. She didn't want to hear it. Whenever I shared my hurt or difficulties from being ridiculed and bullied at school, she would harshly say, "Oh, stop your whining!" Mum had too many of her own struggles to be interested in mine. So, I tried to behave like the daughter she wanted: happy and non-demanding. I focussed on the food I knew she would have waiting for me when we got home.

When we got to the house, I dragged my bag out of the car and went inside to get changed. Mum was waiting with food for me in front of the TV. This day it was an unopened packet of Arnott's Yo-Yo Biscuits. They were yummy, made with sugar, flour, butter, eggs, milk and honey. I dipped them in the tall glass of milk she had poured for me.

Though I was a young teenager, mum spoke and interacted with me like I was a little child. Food was always the mediating factor between us. When she prepared, served or gave me food, it was the closest thing to feeling heard by her. But I had an inner world of ideas, hurts, dreams, and fears that I kept locked up inside. Mum never related to me like I was an equal. I knew I was inferior to her and she was worth more than me. I was to be fed, and to comfort her pain.

Before I had eaten the entire packet of biscuits, mum became angry that I was eating so much and left the room. I finished the packet, and then saw an open bar of chocolate on the lounge room table and ate that. Then I spotted a bag of peanuts and devoured them. The combination of sugar and salt made me thirsty, and I headed to the fridge to gulp down a litre bottle of Coke.

The sugar made me high, lifting my empty and depressed feelings. It was an injection of euphoria in a relentlessly distressing world. But it quickly wore off. I was still hungry—hungry for approval and affirmation, hungry for belonging, hungry to be seen and to know I was worth something, hungry to be loved. Instead, I found a bag of chips in the cupboard and consumed them all.

Mum knew that I was still eating. She called out angrily from the small office, "Jenny, don't eat any more. You won't eat your dinner!"

I stopped eating and turned on the TV to pass the time before dinner, which I immediately started thinking about. This was how most days and evenings went after school. I was hungry, but not for food.

Later in life I realized that mum was a classic enabler. She used food to compensate for the absence of relationship, to pacify my hurts, and get her own fix. Food was the glue that bonded us together. She was happy when she was eating, and I was too.

Mum hated herself, and she hated the reflection of herself in me. My overeating and weight gain were an embarrassment to her, and she was persistent in her jabs and put-downs. She was ashamed of my obesity, and often brought this up in public settings when I was present.

She deflected her own addiction to food by shaming me, yet everyday she packed my lunch with rich food or gave me money to order it. While my classmates ate sandwiches and fruit, I ate a pie and chips. Mum would berate me for being overweight, but each day after school she had cookies, cakes, chips, and lollies ready for me. When I was upset about being bullied and called names by schoolmates, she gave me food.

As long as I was grossly obese, attention was drawn away from her own food and weight problem. Mum could see that my obesity was harming my physical and psychological health. But she needed me to be fat in order to feel better about herself, to escape her misery and distract her from the truth of her own food addiction. Mum abused me with food, just as she did herself. I took it as love. Mum taught me to comfort and protect myself by eating, but I did not realise it was slowly killing me.

When mum was pregnant with me, she developed gestational diabetes. She stayed in the hospital for a week before my birth to control it. Diabetes continued to haunt her for the remainder of her life.

She could not lose weight or control her eating habits. I'm sure the emotional tension and psychological stress she carried contributed to her weight gain as she aged. Instead of facing these issues she blamed her children. More than once she said to me, "I have a big stomach from having you kids!"

In her late forties and fifties, she frequented the local hospital as her doctors sought to slow her degeneration in health. She was prescribed a heavy concoction of medications to control her blood pressure and diabetes. Medical knowledge at the time was limited. Once a patient started on this downward spiral, there was no real answer. Nothing could slow mum's declining condition.

Over time, she developed foot ulcers, and her joints and bones degenerated. She eventually lost sensation in both her feet, and her eyesight failed. She was chronically fatigued and slept on and off throughout the day. Finally, she had a stroke and was never the same person.

Mum's eating issues were the product of her troubled childhood. She had all her bottom teeth removed after high school because she ate sugary food, and her parents could not afford dental care.

Her father was a tormented man who had been the last illegitimate child of a mistress to several men. He lost his mother when he was four years of age and was placed in a boys' home. He married the youngest daughter of the owners of a boarding house where he lived. Working as a carpenter, he struggled to put food on the table.

Mum never spoke well of her father and vowed never to be like him. Her parents separated after she left home, and she often said that she could hear them arguing while she lay in bed at night as a child. Her mother moved in with her son (mum's brother), where she lived until moving to a nursing home a few years before her death.

Her mother was depressed, and about the time of mum's marriage to dad, she tried to hang herself. She was placed in a psychiatric hospital as a result of this. Dad would often remind mum of her mother's failure with, "Stupid bitch! Tried to hang herself by a shoestring to a doorknob!"

To the outside world mum was a capable, intelligent, decent woman with a great sense of humour and a friendly manner. The secretarial skills she learned in the city were valued in our small community. She volunteered her time for the local agricultural society, a local political party, and worked at the town shop to fill in occasionally. But underneath she was cynical, hardened, bitter, and angry with the world.

As a child I walked on eggshells around mum's erratic moods, never knowing when they would turn aggressive and irrational. More than once she told me that she could understand why parents abuse their children. "Sometimes it gets too much, and you just can't control it," she would say.

Like dad, mum was a broken woman. She was hurt and angry with herself, and with the world. Her lack of self-acceptance at the time of my birth was the soil from which our relationship had grown, and she had associated these feelings with me for the rest of her life. Instead of bonding with me, she gave me food.

Overeating was not the root of my weight problem. The misuse of food as a substitute for love was. Mum was a wounded woman and she wounded me. Some of the most painful ways we have been hurt in life are not because we are bad and deserved it, but because others are wounded and act out of it. The most difficult to overcome are those which are caused by the ones we love.

Chapter Five

Can't Remember and Can't Forget

The most devastating wounds of childhood trauma and abuse are not what we remember, but what we block out. There are some experiences in life which we try to hide even from ourselves. We barricade them off from our heart because they are too painful to face. The memories that we banish to the deep shadows of our subconscious, secretly rule and sabotage our lives. They are embedded in our cells and form the core of our self-belief. They fester beneath the surface and become toxic.

One early childhood experience had remained hidden in my subconscious until my late 20s. I was bending over the old cement sink in the laundry, vomiting.

The laundry of the house on the farm had never been renovated. The double cement sink on the wall was supported by two concrete pillars, and an old wringer stood near the window next to it. The taps hanging over the sink were held up by a pipe which carried their water. It was a cold and gloomy room with grey walls and floor.

My stomach was tied in knots, as mum firmly held my head over the sink to prevent my vomit from going everywhere. I could hear the indignation in her voice. She was angry with me. "I don't know what to do with you," she said not knowing why I was vomiting.

I could never remember why I was in the laundry, retching over the cement sink until later in my life. The experiences of childhood sexual abuse were not accessible to my conscious mind as explicit memories. The brain has a survival mechanism that allows one to detach from traumatic events and fragments the memory. Mum always said that kids don't remember their early life, but she was wrong. Though it wasn't until adulthood that I recovered it, my earliest memory was sexual abuse at around 4 years of age. Preschool age (3-5 years) is sadly a common age for this. I have no memory of the perpetrator; I guess I have chosen not to remember.

There were tell-tale signs of my sexual abuse. I was a chronic bed-wetter into my middle childhood years. I was terrified of being alone and the dark. Nightmares tormented my sleep.

Mum would get out of bed and stomp to my room frustrated and angry, "Shut up! You are just imagining things!" She would curse me as I got up, angrily rip off the wet sheet I was laying on and replace it with the drier sheet which had been on top of me. "You woke up because you wet your bed. I don't know what to do with you!"

Most mornings mum would hang the wet sheet on the line without washing it, then put it back on my bed when it dried later in the day. "If you are going to wet your bed all the time, there's no point washing your sheets every day," she complained.

Mum assumed that I wet my bed because I was a bad child, and she blamed it for her stress. Before going to school each day, I stood in front of the heater as she wiped the bottom half of my body with a flannel cloth to wash off the urine. Mum said I stank because I wet my bed. I smelled of stale urine at school, which only gave classmates more ammunition to mock me. In my mind this was further proof that I was a bad and worthless person. Much later in life I discovered that bed-wetting can be a symptom of childhood stress.

I was the youngest of four children. We had photo-albums full of pictures of my siblings in their early years, but very few of me, except a few infant photographs and a couple before starting school. Then, during my school years mum purchased my class photos, almost as compensation for the oversight earlier in my childhood. Later in life I discovered that I was an unwanted child. Mum did not plan to have any more children, especially a girl and was depressed at the time. Dad was sullen upon discovering that he was getting another daughter.

From the first day of my life, I was a nuisance. My older sisters and brother shared a respect for each other and a bond. But there was no such bond with me. I was excluded from their activities. Even in my own family, I never felt that I belonged.

When I was eight, my eldest sister left home. This left an emotional hole in mum's life, which she depended upon me to fill. I could never measure up to my sister in mum's eyes, but I was useful for dumping her emotional burden on, and filling the hole created by her loneliness. She would often complain about dad and lament all her regrets and disappointments. And she would complain about me.

Mum and dad were relieved when I got home from school each day—my mum, because she needed me as an emotional life-preserver and I was a distraction from her mental pain; and my dad, because he didn't want to deal with my mum.

Mum's moods were erratic. She clung to me for relief of her depression and emptiness, but she blamed me for her troubles. Mum swung between nasty and nice, using me as a scapegoat and then offering kindness. She would criticise me relentlessly with comments about my laziness, selfishness and whining, and then she would placate me with sweet words and food. Her emotional swings and criticism left me in constant anxiety. Depending on her mood at the moment, I could be her confidante or scapegoat.

Either way, I concluded I was a bad daughter. For all her criticism of me and emotional dumping, she was never the better for it; I only seemed to exasperate her suffering further. The bond between us was food. We were perfect partners in enabling our emotional eating and food addiction. Food was comfort, it filled the void within us, or so we thought. Whether we were stressed, lonely, exhausted or bored, eating was our first impulse. Mum gave me food as a substitute for love and relationship. And food was mum's way of making up after she hurt me.

We did not eat because we were physically hungry, we were trying to fill an emotional hunger. Emotional hunger requires instant gratification. It craves junk food or sugary snacks that provide an instant rush. Emotional hunger often leads to mindless eating. Before I knew it, I had eaten a whole bag of chips or an entire packet of lollies without really paying attention. My emotional hunger wasn't satisfied once I was full. I kept wanting more and more, often eating until I was uncomfortably stuffed. Emotional hunger left me feeling regret, guilt, and shame.

Mum had two basic modes of relating to me: possessiveness and abandonment. She clung to me when she needed to fill a void, and she blamed me for her misery. There was nothing I wanted more in life than her acceptance, but if it came it never lasted.

I took my emotional hunger and food addiction into adulthood. My solid belief that I was a bad, unlovable, and worthless person was always lurking in the shadows. My failure as a daughter to mum and dad was a dark stain on my soul. As an adult I sought external approval to satiate the internal pain of my parents' indifference and rejection but was suspicious and mistrustful whenever I got it.

So, I ate to fill the void.

I was a larger child at an earlier age than any of my siblings. Dark marks formed around the creases of my neck and around my elbows, because of hormonal changes from weight gain.

It was the kind of food I ate, and the volume of it consumed, that led to my morbid obesity. But it was trauma and shame that was the source of my emotional eating and food addiction. My relationship with food became a vicious cycle: I was bad and so I overate. I overate and I was bad. I was depressed and so I overate. I overate and I was depressed. I was the problem-child to my parents and so I overate. I overate and was the problem-child. I was emotionally exhausted and so I overate. I overate and I was emotionally exhausted.

Sorting all this out later in life was not an easy task. The physiological and psychological reasons that drove my increase in weight were complex. On top of the sexual abuse, toxic family relationships, and genetics, I was also living in a society that judged obese people. The common myth that a person is obese simply because they lack the motivation and willpower to stop overeating, is complete ignorance of the factors that contribute to obesity.

As a consequence of my childhood sexual abuse, I shut down my sexuality and closed myself off from warmth or affection, especially by men. Choosing to ignore the greatest trauma of my childhood, led to a lack of connection with myself and others because of my shame. Connection is how we experience love, but I walled myself off from others. Instead, I ate. We all have misplaced dependencies to fill a void that only love, and connection can fill. Mine was food.

Obesity put my entire family in a vulnerable position. Eventually, each of us would succumb to one, if not all, of the degenerative diseases associated with obesity such as cancer, diabetes, kidney disease, osteoarthritis, high blood pressure and high cholesterol. I was classified as morbidly obese as a child, which did not bode well for my adulthood. Attempts at weight loss never worked. I was not in a good place for a healthy future.

Psychologist Carl Jung wrote, "I am not what happened to me, I am what I choose to become." Weight gain was the result of what happened to me. However, I could not live my life as a victim. Instead, I learned to overcome the consequences of abuse and find my way out of it. I can never undo what was done to me. But I disentangled the shame and fear that governed my life and drove my self-sabotaging beliefs and behaviours. It was not easy; it was often hell! Was it worth it? Yes.

No one would argue that the circumstances I grew up in were unfair. But bitterness and anger did not give me freedom and health. Those who hurt me were ultimately not my problem. The web of wounds inside myself, were my responsibility as an adult. Remaining a victim would not have given me freedom. There was love for me, just as there is for everyone. The challenge was to discover that I was loved, and to love myself enough to find a way out of the pain.

Chapter Six

Three Hundred Pounds Plus Twelve

Sitting with my legs crossed on my small grey mat on the classroom floor, I was spellbound by my teacher. Her hair was done in the beehive style of the sixties, wound from the nape of her neck to a peak at the top of her head. She wore a short skirt and high heels. I gazed at her in awe, mesmerized by her beauty. She was the prettiest woman I had ever seen. Mum usually wore a plain pinafore with an apron over the top.

The teacher had told us to bring a small mirror so that we could see ourselves mouthing vowels. I watched as she mouthed "e", then did the same into my mirror. When the lesson was finished, she told us to return to our desks.

Quickly hopping up from the floor, all the other kids scurried to their seats. I was much slower. It was a struggle to push myself off the floor and get to my feet. I was the biggest child in the room, even eclipsing the older students in a combined class of different grades.

Then the teacher who I adored yelled out, "Look at the big gorilla get off the floor!" The classroom erupted in laughter, and my heart withered in shame as I slowly walked back to my desk, hanging my head.

School was excruciating, trying to make it to the final bell in fear of bullying and rejection. I was grossly overweight, had body odour, and sores under the folds of my skin. More than once I wet my pants during class.

I cried a lot at school. By my second year of primary school I was around the 130-pound (60 kg) mark. Sometimes we had school nurses visit, which I dreaded. The class teacher weighed each student in preparation. When I stepped onto the scales, the other kids watched and laughed.

Making friends was near impossible. I was avoided by the other students. I was socially inept, and during recess and lunch while the other kids played, I sat at a distance by myself.

In the fourth grade our school went on an excursion. This involved walking less than a mile to a scenic area. I walked with an awkward waddle. Not able to keep up with my grade, I was told to walk with the littlest kids, which I towered over like a mammoth. I was exhausted and fell behind. The teachers nagged me to walk faster.

When we made it near a large picturesque pond, I could walk no further. The rest of my classmates enjoyed the view while I sat down beside the car of the school secretary, totally spent. My only friend, a girl in my class with a disability, was sitting in the back seat. She rolled down her window and said, "Mrs Jones reckons you should be made to walk. She said you are too fat and need some exercise. She reckons your parents should put you on a diet." Exhausted, my class teacher had to take me back to school in her car.

PE classes were horrifying. Once trying to do a long jump, I fell heavily on my right leg and suffered a severe knee sprain. Obesity caused my legs to turn outward, which was not suitable for jumping. The teacher gave me little sympathy. Although I loved swimming, exposing my legs was humiliating. I could barely see my knees under the fat, and my legs rubbed together. The kids teased me and called me a whale as I entered the water.

Dentist appointments were long gruelling affairs. My mouth was a battleground. A typical appointment lasted well over an hour to complete the fillings. I did not fit easily into the chair, and I left with a stiff jaw filled with metal. My dentist was an older, gruff man with fingers which tasted of cigars. It was obvious to him that my teeth were decayed because of the food I ate. On one visit he asked, "How much do you weigh?" I stammered, "I don't talk about my personal issues." As he turned his head to look at the dental nurse, I saw an expression of mockery on his face.

By the final year of primary school, I had reached 300 pounds (132 kg). I was twelve years old. The Education Department sent a health nurse to our school. Each visit to our class, she would ask me to leave the room with her so she could check my weight and speak privately to me about my weight problem. To my embarrassment, I was escorted out in front of all the other students.

During her visits she asked me a series of questions including what I ate, if I understood how obese I was, how long I'd been this way, what we ate at home, and if my mum was overweight. Feeling ashamed of my weight and overeating, I denied that there was a problem, but she called mum to come to school so my weight could be discussed. This created conflict between my parents and led to arguments. I wanted to be left alone. Food was the only thing that kept me together. It was my way of receiving love, and what kept mum and me together. She recommended that I change my eating habits, and I felt the only security I had was about to be ripped away.

The news that I had reached 300 pounds was somehow discovered by a few kids and it spread throughout the entire school. The cruelty and bullying intensified.

My skin turned into rolls, which hung over my abdomen, waist and back. My arms and legs grew in circumference. I developed ulcers from the excess fat and skin under my armpits, in my groin, and under each of the rolls. They bled so heavily that when I had my first period, I mistook it for a burst ulcer. My legs chafed, which also caused rashes and fungal infections. The skin infections smelled, making me self-conscious.

When I left primary school, the headmaster wrote in my report that he was concerned about my weight and its effect on my relationships with my peers. His recommendation to mum and dad was that I attend a residential weight loss camp. He said that I was an intelligent girl, and missing school for up to six months would not impact my education. My parents were furious. They were not interested in dealing with their own bad eating patterns, much less mine.

Mum and dad were ashamed of my weight, but they also ignored it. I know underneath they felt responsible but were not willing to admit it. According to dad, I lacked willpower.

High school was worse. A group of students would walk arm-in-arm across the school yard yelling "Gigantor!" One of their favourite names for me was "Jenworth", named after the Kenworth semi-trailer. During the late '70s there was a popular song called "Marshall's Portable Music Machine". The kids enjoyed changing the words to "Marshall's Portable Blubber Machine".

One of my teachers would make a grunting sound, accentuating my heaviness as I stepped onto the school bus to go home each afternoon. One of the kids sitting beside me on the bus would draw a line in chalk down the middle of our seat to indicate that I took up more than my share. Like a turtle, I would withdraw myself into my shell for protection. But even this provided little relief because of the shame and self-hatred that ambushed my own mind.

Occasionally there was a teacher who tried to reach out to me, but I was too afraid and ashamed to accept it. I spent most of my school days alone, often in the library or lunch shed. Mum sewed my school uniforms because they were not made for my size. She hated sewing and let me know about it and would complain about my obesity from behind the sewing machine. I myself despised sewing. In school sewing classes I was too large to create clothes from a pattern. Mum would increase the pattern by adding a seam to it, which annoyed the teacher because it threw everything off.

I excelled in my maths and science classes. The black and white nature of these subjects suited me well. Numbers, equations, and the systematic structure of science tracked easily with my brain. But more abstract subjects in the humanities like literature, art, history, politics, or religion were a different story. These required deeper thought, introspection, and expression of my own opinions. I had no confidence in my thoughts and was petrified of speaking in front of others.

My final year in high school I chose high-end maths, physics, chemistry and English, known as the "suicide five". I had no idea what I wanted to do with my life. Planning for my future was not on the top of my mind, surviving each day was. My cousin was an accountant, I was good with numbers, and dad said accounting would make a lot of money, so I chose to train as an accountant.

Mum's health deteriorated during my school years. She had numerous stays in the hospital because of high blood pressure and put on heavy medication to manage it. The medication slowed her down, but dad accused her of being lazy and having no willpower.

This was the beginning of mum's serious and rapid decline. Her diabetes worsened. She once had been a red-faced, stressed and moody person, now she was fatigued and depressed. Mum was not able to lose weight, and her interest in life was all but gone. She was easily overwhelmed and during the day she napped on and off. Her community involvement had stopped long ago.

Mum and dad's marriage hit another low. Dad went to bed early to avoid dealing with mum and did not speak to her at breakfast. At dinner, he would either belittle mum or give her the cold shoulder.

Mum was lonely and desperate for company. It was a lonely life being sick on a farm in a sparsely populated area. She found comfort in music, using it to soothe her soul, but dad had no patience for it. If a record was playing when he was home, he would lash out at her, "Kick that bloody thing in the guts!"

My heart ached for mum. I carried her unhappiness and even felt responsible for it. I feared her depression, and it left me in a state of anxiety. I was engulfed in her pain. Some days she would desperately cling to me like I was her only reason for living, other days she would withdraw entirely, and I felt abandoned and alone. The good days were when mum needed me and she would hug me on the old couch at the back of the house. We were emotionally dependent on each other, but I needed her more than she needed me.

Food remained my way of easing my emptiness. My obesity made my life increasingly difficult. Making my bed was exhausting. Climbing two or three steps at a time was a challenge. The simplest task winded me. I had difficulty walking and trouble breathing.

A 12-year-old girl's weight is usually between 68 and 135 pounds (45 kg). I weighed 300 (132 kg). Most kids my age rode bikes, climbed trees, jumped rope, and went to community events with friends and family. But my life was spent alone and consumed by self-hatred. I was the problem child. I wasn't worthy to be loved.

So, I ate.

Chapter Seven
You Never Leave Home

A few days before I turned 21, my family was invited to the party of a former school classmate of mine, who was also celebrating his 21st birthday. During the celebration, his mother asked me to come forward. She explained that she knew mum was ill and was not able to prepare a birthday cake, so she had made one for me. The cake was decorated in white royal icing, purple decorations, gold candles, and "Happy Birthday Jenny" in pretty purple letters.

Embarrassed, I slowly walked up to receive the cake and thanked her for the kind and thoughtful gesture. This caring act stood in contrast to the heartache that surrounded my birthday.

On the eve of turning 21, mum was back in the hospital. Her blood sugar was high, and there were ulcers on her feet that would not heal. She was not aware of the problem at first because her feet had grown numb, all symptoms of diabetes.

The country doctor did all he could to help her body heal. He lowered mum's sugar levels and elevated her feet. These measures had little effect and he decided to do a skin graft. The surgery was scheduled for the day of my birthday.

On the morning of the surgery mum broke down. She was not one to show emotions in public, but she was at the end of herself. The hospital rang dad to notify him of the ordeal. In her conversation with dad, mum told him that she wanted to spend the birthday with her 'baby'. She felt terrible about my birthday, and guilty that my friend's mother had baked me a birthday cake; she was a bad mother.

When dad hung up the phone he was in tears. Dad insisted that he, along with my sister and I go to the hospital to calm her down. My sister decided that we would take lunch to the hospital and eat it with mum to cheer her up, and to take the cake along with us. This was the way my family showed love and care, with food.

It was deeply disappointing to celebrate one of the biggest milestones of my life in this way. I tried my best to hide my feelings but made the mistake of telling my sister I was upset. She responded by saying, "You only think of yourself, Jennifer! How do you think I feel? I have to make lunch and take it over there!"

My 21st birthday was a mixture of toxic emotions. I was scared that mum was sick. I felt guilty that I had added to mum's distress. I was hurt that my special day was focussed on mum. Feelings of shame tormented me for thinking this way, and for being the selfish person everyone said I was. I felt anger, but I didn't know who or what to be angry with except myself. I was always the problem.

We packed the car with lunch and the uncut 21st birthday cake made for me, and we drove to the hospital. When we arrived, mum's face was red from tears, but she was relieved to see us. She wished me happy birthday, as did the nurses. We lit the candles, sang, and cut the cake.

The thick sugary icing on my piece of cake gave me a moment of euphoria, but it did not ease my emotional pain. I knew that the focus had to be on making mum happy. Resentment welled up inside me as I remembered how we celebrated my sister's 21st birthday at a fancy restaurant.

I came to realize that the real problem was never the day of my birthday. It was deeper than that. Being born was the real problem. My life was a mistake. As an unwanted child, I was the problem. This was true of every day; birthdays only served to put a spotlight on the whole issue.

My 21st birthday fell during my second year of university. I was studying for a degree in accounting. Living away from the stress and turmoil of home improved my academic performance. It was easier to focus.

However, my eating and weight problems continued. Hair was growing on my chin as the fat cells created testosterone. The dark stains around my elbows, neck, and other parts of my body had worsened due to hormonal changes. My obesity had severely affected my posture. I developed an outward curvature of the spine, which caused me to walk hunchbacked.

Living away from my parents meant I could eat whatever and whenever I wanted, without anyone looking over my shoulder. I sewed my own clothes in order to have outfits to wear. It was humiliating that I could not fit in many of the lecture hall seats or chairs. I often improvised to make it work. When I found a seat in which I could fit, I would beeline toward it at the start of class. If it was already taken, I'd be seized with anxiety.

Overall, the environment at university seemed more accepting. I formed a close friendship with another student in my first year. She was more confident than me and I always felt inferior. When I would visit her parent's home, we had long conversations about my family, which felt cathartic.

Verbal presentations at my university were excruciating. I hated people looking at me. Being morbidly obese, I felt like the object of judgment and disgust. No one judged me more than myself. But this was the reality of life as an obese person—the looks, the laughs, the whispers.

On campus I became involved in a group of Christian international students. They were an accepting and friendly lot, and love and grace seemed to be their central teachings. One of them invited me to attend their Pentecostal church. That was an adventure! Healings, visions, prophecies, and visitations from the Holy Spirit were regularly reported. I even managed to speak in tongues. It was new and exciting at first but was not ultimately satisfying or life-altering. The simple love and acceptance I received from that group of students was worth more to me than a thousand Sundays of ecstatic utterances.

Although it was good to be many miles separated from my parents and the family farm, I learned that I never really "left home". My wounds, self-hatred, food addiction, and weight travelled with me everywhere I went. The coping mechanism I had learned was to soothe my emotional hurt and anxiety with eating. Food was a dependable and unconditional source of comfort. Food was impartial. Food was love.

My 21st birthday was not a happy one. I sat in the hospital eating cake with mum to make her feel happy. Food can distract you from your pain but cannot take away your pain. There is no piece of cake that can do that.

Chapter Eight

The Graduation Photo That Never Happened

In my final year of university mum had a stroke. She was only 57 years old, but her body and mind had significantly deteriorated because of her diabetes. Her memory was worsening, and the nerve endings in her feet were damaged. She spent much of the day in the house with her legs up. Mum was in and out of the local hospital with ulcers on her legs and feet caused by poor circulation. Finally, she fell extremely ill in the local hospital and was rushed by ambulance to the city. She was diagnosed with blood poisoning known as septicaemia. The infection had spread throughout her body. Overnight she suffered a stroke.

It was late January during university holidays, and I was home on the farm. Dad walked through the kitchen door of our house, his face lined with fear and tears running down his cheeks. "Your mother's had a stroke" he said in a distressed voice. And then added, "It's as bad as Mrs Smith's" to give weight to the announcement. Mrs Smith had a stroke years earlier which left her unable to speak and in a wheelchair.

As the day unfolded and we were given more information, it was obvious that mum would never be the same again. Her heart was damaged from the complications of her diabetes. The stroke occurred in the right side of her brain. She could no longer walk or control the left side of her body. Her mouth was numb, and she was unable to feed herself.

I drove back to the city to see her in hospital but was unprepared for the complete change of her personality. The first words she said to me were, "Hello dear", words I had never heard mum speak before. Her appearance, demeanour, language—this was not the mother I had known for 22 years. "Mum," I said, wanting to relate as we would normally, "would you like me to get something for you?" "Whatever dear", was her response.

Whatever connection we previously had was now nothing more than a memory. But each night I travelled across the city to the hospital to sit with mum, hoping she would return to the woman she had once been. Instead, she was digressing into a child. The smallest annoyance sent her into a temper tantrum and tears. At other times she was depressed and bemoaned how miserable and hopeless life was and would start sobbing.

When mum returned home from the hospital, she evolved into a giggly, silly adolescent. She was self-absorbed and dressed like a teenager. She lost her inhibitions and made inappropriate comments to visitors or those she saw in public. Doctors had weighed the possibility of her needing psychiatric care but decided to wait and see how her condition progressed. People were shocked and putt-off by mum's behaviour.

As disturbing as it was to see mum operating with no filter, I wasn't as startled as others. Over the years, mum had expressed privately to me many of her severe and bitter views of life, of others. But seeing her freely spew all this out was mortifying.

I struggled to complete my final year of university, and my grades dropped considerably. It was a demanding year balancing my studies and tending to mum. I coped by deluding myself into believing that my relationship with her would return to normal. As dysfunctional as this "normal" had been, it was familiar. I was thoroughly entrenched in co-dependence with mum. There was no delineation of where I stopped, and she began. She was emotionally abusive but because it was attention, I took it as love. My life was mum and food. Now there was no mum, which meant it was necessary to eat more to fill the void.

Mum could no longer remember when I was born, how old I was, or that I was in university. She forgot all my likes and dislikes. It wasn't lost on me that she seemed to have far better recollection when it came to my older brother and sisters. Then one day out of nowhere, when I was alone with her, she said, "I'm glad I had you now dear." This was the first time I had ever heard her say anything about how she felt about my birth. As I turned this over in my mind, her words became more troubling. Apparently, she had never wanted me, and it took a stroke to bring this to the surface.

It wasn't just mum who was going through massive adjustments to life after her stroke, the entire dynamics of our family changed. Dad and my siblings pulled together to care for mum, but I was left out. Everyone's place in the family was determined by what role they were playing to help mum, but I was pushed to the side with no role at all. When I asserted myself to ask what I could do, it was met by accusations of selfishness and laziness, and that I could not be depended upon to take any responsible role with mum. Whenever I tried to be useful, it was mocked and belittled. The family would discuss and make major decisions about mum's health, but I was never involved.

Dad turned over the management of the family finances to my brother. He decided that I should no longer be receiving any financial assistance from the family for my university expenses. Instead, he told me I'd have to get a job. He also took it upon himself to calculate how much my parents had spent on my university degree and angrily told me how much it had cost them. It was as if I was a criminal.

When I spoke with mum about it, she responded, "They're doing a lot for me dear." And then in a mocking tone said, "Boo hoo, I'm going to cry too!" She told me, "Your studies are selfish! It doesn't help me at all. I'm the sick one!" I never asked for anything again from mum or dad.

I felt like a piece of driftwood, unmoored in the world. Ostracized and abandoned by my family, I was forced to face the world alone. My mind became a battleground, filled with explosive thoughts. My family's rejection triggered the long-forgotten memories of being abused as a child. I played over in my head my relationship with mum and realized it had been a farce.

For the first time in my life I was faced with the ugly reality of my existence. I was not meant to be here. My conception was an accident, and my birth a curse. Dad despised me and I had suffered his psychological abuse. Mum regretted me, and I was the victim of her emotional incest. From the first day of my life, I was the unwelcome intrusion, problem child and fat daughter, who was not worthy of love.

Even with the stress at home, and the demands of my final year of university, I passed all my subjects and completed my degree. On the day of graduation, I was excited, yet grief stricken. As I walked into the theatre with my graduating class, I looked out at the sea of unfamiliar faces. When my name was called, I climbed the steps onto the stage to receive my degree. Out of the corner of my eye, I could see mum in the aisle in her wheelchair with dad and my eldest sister sitting beside her in their seats. She was waving her arms madly like a small child to get my attention. I could faintly hear her yelling, "Hello dear!"

After the ceremony, pictures were taken of graduates with their parents and families. I searched for mum and dad, but they were nowhere to be found. I had my graduation picture taken without them.

When I got home, I asked disappointingly why they were not there after the graduation for the photo. My sister was furious and reprimanded me about how selfish and ungrateful I was. She said that mum had been cold, so they left early. I felt ashamed of myself. I was crushed and wished I had never attended my graduation.

I learned in my family that I had no right to have my own needs and feelings or depend on anyone for anything. Life revolved around mum and dad's unhappiness and suffering. Somehow, I was the one to blame, until I was sufficiently trained to blame myself. It was no longer necessary for others to condemn me. I had locked myself into a prison cell of hatred and threw away the key.

I sometimes wonder what it would have felt like to have a mother and father who were proud of me, saw good in me, and believed in me. I can't imagine what it would be like to have a father who was my pillar, protector, and defender; or a mother who cherished and nurtured me; or siblings with whom I was close, and who always had my back.

I would have given anything for just one moment of feeling special to mum and dad. My life had been lived with a hunger for their affirmation and love. Instead, I was left to appease this hunger with food. I discovered that chocolate cake and chips could serve as a substitute for love, provide temporary relief from my pain and make me happy.

After university, I packed my bags, left home, and was tossed in the lion's den of something commonly referred to as "adulthood." It was time to take my obese self into the real world. With no self-confidence, full of shame and self-hatred, I would be entering the workforce and facing the trials of independence.

Pulling out of the farm driveway felt like an escape, and when the house was out of view, I nervously let out a sigh of relief. Leaving home held the promise of a fresh start.

My newfound sense of freedom quickly dissolved into panic and dread. I tried calming myself by reasoning. Afterall, how could life get any worse?

I was about to find out.

Chapter Nine

Fat Girls Don't Get Promoted

"Jenny, I need some help?", a student called from the other side of the room. "Coming" I said, as I made my way to her desk. We were studying maths, which is a subject many people hate. But I love maths!

One of the biggest obstacles to students is the belief they are "not good at maths." Maths is not a talent that everyone has. However, it can be learned. Some people have a true love for it and excel in it, but any person is capable of learning basic maths.

This student was able to master the maths I was teaching. But she was hindered by her limiting belief about herself. I explained the concept I had presented earlier in class, and we worked through the problems until she got it. I had her work it out for herself with a few exercises until it was clear for her. My goal is always for the student to experience success at maths and gain confidence in their ability.

I turned from her desk and addressed the rest of the class, "You can pass this subject. You can succeed at maths! You only lack confidence. It takes time but you can do it. If you have any questions, please ask me. I am here to help you. I want to help you learn. That is why I am here."

At the end of the class I packed up my computer and folders and headed to my other job. When I arrived, I had to re-focus. It was the end of the financial year, and I had begun preparation of the financial statements for the Annual General Meeting. My emails were full of other issues, and staff came into my office to discuss their work.

I enjoyed my mix of work, teaching at the local university, and accounting for small organizations. At each of these jobs I felt valued and needed. But it was not this way when I first entered the workforce. Like those students, I had my own crisis of self-confidence and many self-limiting beliefs. Unfortunately, there was no one to help or encourage me. However, there were plenty of people to inhibit my success.

Finding a job when I was morbidly obese with no self-confidence was a nightmare. Prospective employers were thrilled with my resume, but this excitement quickly changed when they met me in person at interviews. In every interview it was obvious that my weight made me unattractive. My obesity meant I was lazy, unmotivated, irresponsible, inept, unsightly and dumb.

Eventually I found employment with a small business in a town about three hours distance from where I grew up. I found a small flat to live in, signed a lease agreement, and set up my utilities. All my possessions in the world consisted of a car, and the personal belongings I managed shove into it.

The thought of earning my own money and having my own life felt good. It was freeing to live out from under my parents' control and the toxicity of family dynamics. It also meant there was no one to monitor or prevent my overeating. I no longer had to sneak food and hide eating. I could eat whatever I wanted, as much as I wanted, whenever I wanted.

This was all too good to be true.

My first day on the job was a rude awakening, and the trauma I once endured at home was now replaced by the same at work. My starting salary was identical to the young man who started with me, but he did not have an accounting degree. The managers treated me with the same contempt dad did. It became clear that the work environment was toxic with misogyny, narcissism, bullying, verbal and emotional abuse. And I was a fat female, lowest on the pecking order.

Having no self-confidence, I dutifully accepted the demeaning way I was treated. Afterall, I was an accidental and unwelcome intrusion into the world who deserved such treatment. The situation at work so perfectly mirrored the dynamics of my home, that I just picked up where I left off. From the start, I believed I was a failure. I was fortunate and indebted to these people for offering me a job, given that I was inferior to them. Any criticism aimed at me was deserved.

I could not bring myself to call the managers by their first name as my co-workers did. Instead, I used 'Mr.' and their surname. I was an outcast in the office and spent my lunches alone.

One of the senior managers took great delight in finding fault with my work. I was constantly questioning myself, which hindered my productivity. He called me into his office one evening when we were alone in the building. "Jenny, what is this?" he said, pointing to the work I had done for him. He glared at me in a long disapproving silence and then erupted, "What am I supposed to do with this?!"

Of course, he had not made clear to me the details I needed to complete the work as he wanted.

"I don't know what to do with you, Jenny", he continued with his lashing. "Stacy doesn't have a degree and she works just as fast as you." Stacy was the unqualified, attractive, slim, young blonde girl that all the men gawked over. "I think you are tired," he said as he looked my obese body up and down.

On another occasion, staff were asked to attend a professional development program at a venue away from work. Despite my fear of further rejection, I gave in and decided to attend. After the evening session a staff member and I chose to share a dessert in the resort restaurant. Mr. Johnson came walking in and yelled out, "Jenny! Why are you eating that?" He came up to our table and continued his demeaning comments. "Have you got your pretty dress on, Jenny?" he said sarcastically.

Every day at work I felt judged and mocked. I sometimes caught the looks of disgust and scorn behind my back. There always seemed to be something I was doing wrong.

But the truth is, the work I was hired to do was usually done well. As an obese person I had learned there was little margin for error, and I was obsessively thorough and meticulous to avoid any further rejection. Despite this, I was never acknowledged for the good work I did. Because everyone saw the office managers belittle and demean me, I had little respect from the other staff.

Over time, I became obsessive about my mistakes. I wanted to avoid the criticism from Mr. Johnson in particular. But this reduced my productivity, as I took longer to complete tasks. I was then hauled over the coals for taking too long.

The dynamics in the office was so stressful that I vomited each day before going into work. I wasn't angry at them. I was angry at me. The abuse I endured was deserved. I was not thin and attractive like Stacy, confident and self-assured like Marie, or energetic and vivacious like Teresa. I was fat and worthless Jenny. Every evening I would walk out the door, hating myself more than the day before. My only consolation was knowing that a jar of peanut butter and a loaf of bread were awaiting me at home.

My pay rate increased very little over time. Eventually, I discovered that it was the same as the unqualified female staff who answered the phones and did the bidding of our office managers, despite my qualifications and level of work. One day I was asked to answer phones, and from then on, I was expected to answer them regularly. This increased my workload significantly, but I was constantly grilled over how long I took to complete my work.

When it was time for my performance review, I was called into Mr. Johnson's office where he and one of the younger managers were waiting for me. They closed the door, and I was given a form which scored my performance. My quality of work was marked as poor. Stunned, I asked how this could be. I was told, "We are having problems with your handwriting!" I was also too slow. My morale also received a low score. When I asked about the high-end work I had completed, they looked at each other with blank stares, and the younger manager muttered that it was fine.

One afternoon the managers called me into a meeting. When I walked into the room, the men were all sitting around the conference table. They asked me how I thought I was performing in my position. I told them that I believed my work was good, but this was refuted by Mr. Johnson who reminded me of a name I had misspelled on a file. They pressured me to resign and indicated they were prepared to fire me if I didn't. I agreed. Turns out that they had already found someone to replace me.

Weight discrimination has always been a socially acceptable injustice. Research shows that weight-based stigma, prejudice and discrimination are rampant. These biases often translate into mistreatment of people. There are significant penalties for people who are overweight or obese at every step of the employment process: hiring, evaluations, promotion and firing.

Most employers would rather choose a potential employee who is of normal weight than someone who is visibly overweight. Obese women earn less per year than those at a normal weight. Many employers believe that the cause of obesity is poor life choices, and that it is preventable and can be overcome with willpower.

As an obese person I was belittled. Few really knew or cared to know my story and who I was. Everything they needed to know was visible; I was morbidly obese. They did not take the time to get to know me or understand my history, and how food was the only way that I knew how to cope.

During this season of my life I longed for someone to feel my hurt and understand my pain. People told me that I should stop eating, but they were not willing to understand what it was like for a piece of chocolate cake to be the only thing I had to save me from myself.

I have learned not to judge people but to understand them. Being judged is one of the most painful human experiences. Judgement is rejection when we most need acceptance, love and compassion. We quickly turn into life coaches when it comes to the problems and imperfections of others.

One of our greatest needs as human beings is to be seen, and to know that we are worthy and deserving of love just the way we are. Nowadays I take every opportunity to tell people how good and special they are because I know how much it means to me.

Chapter Ten

When Mum Died

Walking in after lunch that afternoon, one of the reception staff informed me about my eldest sister's call.

"Jenny, your sister phoned. She wants you to call back."

I knew straight away that something was wrong. My family never rang me at work. The receptionist added, "She sounded upset."

I went directly to my office to phone her back. She answered in a distressed voice and barely got the two words out before she began to sob, "Mum's dead."

When we had finished speaking, I hung up the phone and sobbed loudly. It had been 5 years since mum's stroke. I was now living on my own, but my unhealed wounds were running my life. Co-dependent beliefs and behaviour die hard.

I still carried the painful feeling of being unworthy and flawed. I felt useless, taking up people's time and wasting space in the world. I blamed myself for every personal struggle, and believed I deserved the abuse I suffered from others. The constant fear of rejection hung over my head, and I withdrew from people as much as possible, living as a recluse. I was lonely and depressed.

If mum was alive, there was always a faint flicker of hope that I would receive her approval and be the cherished daughter she wanted. But now that flicker had been snuffed out. Mum was dead.

As I drove the three hours back to the farm, conflicting emotions raged within me. Before mum's death, my family had rarely contacted me except to criticize me for not returning home more often to help care for her. Every two weeks I had headed back to the family farm and received a lashing for not doing my part. Once dad phoned me and was irate, "You selfish bitch! Your mother nearly died last night, and you didn't come home." Meanwhile, I was doing all I could to hold down my job in a state of deep depression.

Eventually, I gave up and returned every 5 weeks at most. Visiting so regularly did nothing for my reputation in the family, and whatever I offered was met with indifference.

After mum's stroke, I had not been included in any discussions about her health, or any decisions about her care. She was never happy with what I did for her and complained that I did not do enough. She was indifferent and callous toward me. I could not work out what I had done wrong but blamed myself, nonetheless. The year before she died, I was at a breaking point. I was consumed with guilt about living away from home, even though I had been pushed to leave. Once I was gone, she no longer had any use for me. It was as if I had been disposed of like a piece of rubbish.

About an hour from home, these feelings converged into anger. My childhood and youth were spent bearing the burden of mum's unhappiness. Now living on my own, I was spending tremendous emotional energy denying the reality of her rejection, telling myself that she had really loved me, and that I had misunderstood her motivations. The psychological contortions I performed in my mind were exhausting. The emotional energy expended left very little for my own life. The futility of trying to please mum had destroyed my self-worth and left me with a food addiction that was sabotaging my life and health as a woman.

But despite all this, mum's death was deeply distressing. I loved her, and that would never change. All the childhood suffering didn't erase the raw reality that I had lost my mother—the mother who delivered me into existence, gave me a name, occupied the centre of my world, and got me into adulthood. Mum's death meant grieving the reality of her absence, surrendering any remaining hope of gaining her love, and letting go of the relationship I had hoped for.

As I pulled onto the farm driveway and drove toward the house, I knew from the cars parked that both my sisters were there. This meant that everyone in my immediate family would be waiting. My stomach was in knots at the thought of facing them.

When I walked in the door, something felt different. Dad, my brother and sisters were sitting around the kitchen table with grave faces. For a few moments, sorrow had created a spirit of tenderness and harmony between us.

On the day of the funeral, dad wanted me beside him in the car on the drive to the church. "You were her youngest child," he said. Reluctantly, I pleased him and sat at his side in the back of the car.

A friend, Bill, was the minister who officiated mum's funeral. He was kind to mum's memory, speaking of her as a woman of virtue and strength. He droned on about mum's perfections. But this was not the mother that I knew. Confusion and guilt intensified within me. Maybe it was true after all, and I was deluded.

Mum's body was taken away and cremated. Her ashes were returned to the family farm where they sat on a shelf in the bedroom where my sisters and I slept. After a few months we decided to bury them at the local cemetery. At the spot, my brother took his shovel and dug a hole. He dropped the urn into it and filled it with dirt. "Bye mum", he said, his eyes moist with sadness. It was a sombre moment until my sister suddenly grabbed our arms, pulled us together over the burial spot, and said, "She was a bitch, but I loved her!"

I forced myself to get back into my life, but I felt like an emotional zombie with an unrelenting emptiness inside. As dysfunctional as it had been, the fact remained that my life had always revolved around mum. Without her, I felt lost. I slumped deeper into depression. Reluctantly, I visited a doctor who recommended that I take two weeks of sick leave. When I presented the doctor's note to my manager at work, he questioned its validity and I was criticized about the money it would cost for me to take leave, "You need to sort your head out! I'm paying for this!" I took the two weeks but was tormented by guilt over the expense to my workplace.

My weight ballooned as I grieved mum's death. There was no amount of food that could fill the gaping whole inside. I ate my way through the pain of her death and was quickly approaching 600 pounds (250 kg).

One of my few friends at the time was Scott, who ran a small car repair shop. He was a down to earth, kind and accepting soul. From the conversations we had, I discovered that he had his own tortured childhood and youth. I felt at ease to share with him my own grief, and he listened with compassion and understanding.

The sound of an open fire could be heard from the back of his workshop. It was made from an old brake drum. Scott would push wood offcuts into the fire and sometimes ask me to hold the longer pieces until they could be pushed in entirely. The crackling sound of burning wood relaxed me. I sat on an old swivel seat beside the fire and talked about work and my family. He offered me lollies as he worked. Scott was a ray of light in an otherwise dark and lonely world.

But as time marched on, I found I could not escape the emptiness I felt from mum's death. A mother never really dies; we never stop loving our mother. We never forget her. But mum would always be dead. Nobody could make that right. We can't be protected from our suffering. Tears can't wash it away. Food can't comfort it away. It's just there, and we have to survive it.

My mum's death was the worst thing that had ever happened to me. I needed help to keep afloat and not be pulled under by my grief and depression.

I turned to the church in the hope of God's support.

Chapter Eleven

God Hates Obese People

Singing with the rest of the congregation at the fundamentalist church I attended was comforting and gave me reprieve from my emotional turmoil. I found refuge in singing with all my heart. It was like entering another world where I felt no pain. The simple songs opened within me feelings of beauty, love, and belonging. In those moments I touched something that was bigger than myself, calming my inner turmoil, and lifting me out of my pain and suffering.

But my pain would return when the music stopped. Inevitably, someone would give "a word from the Lord", and I would brace myself for the heaviness of the message. One Sunday, a visiting preacher called for people who were struggling in their life to come forward for prayer. I responded by walking toward the pulpit expecting compassion and understanding for my depression. When I reached the front of the church, he "laid hands on me" and with a booming voice for all the church to hear, yelled out, "I rebuke these lusts of the flesh! Oh Lord, help this woman with her lusts of the flesh!"

I was horrified! God had announced my "sin" to everyone. It was plain to see that I was obese, but now it was official—being fat was a lack of faith and stained the reputation of God.

But I knew that being obese was bad. My childhood and youth had left me with no doubt about that. All religion did was put sophisticated theological terms on my condition like "depraved" and "sin" and added God to the list of those who condemned me. I spent every day of my life knowing I was a failure to my earthly father, only to discover I was a disappointment to my heavenly father too.

Me and church were like oil and water. Firstly, I swore. I was born into an expletive throwing family and four-letter words were part of my regular vocabulary. Second, I had my own views. This did not go well in an environment where independent thinking was a sin. Thirdly, I had no filter. I was hopelessly incapable of faking my true thoughts and feelings. Neither did people get my dry sense of humour. Fourth, I was too much into love. What drew me to church was hearing so many people speak of the "love of God" and how it had changed their lives. But at this church, God's love was less important than church attendance, tithing, correct theology, obeying God's commands, submission to church leaders, tithing, self-denial, walking the straight and narrow, steering clear of unbelievers and the carnalities of the world, and … tithing.

I managed to find a few other wounded oddballs and outcasts at the church, and we flocked together like birds of a feather. They accepted my foul language, brazen honesty, and quirky sense of humour. This small tribe of people were "church" to me.

But despite this little group, my involvement was becoming increasingly bad for my mental and physical health. Before I knew it, I was attending twice every Sunday and practically whenever the doors were open for programs and events. The freedom of living on my own had been usurped by the demands of godliness. I gave up my worldly ways, and listened only to Christian music, reading Christian books, and socializing with Christian people. My life became church.

I swallowed shame-based religion. The message was loud and clear: I was nothing without God. I did not deserve God and was not worthy of His love. Sunday sermons told me I was born with a spiritual disease, and that God looked upon me as a "filthy rag". I went to church in search of a God of love, and instead found one who condemned me to eternal conscious torment because I was human.

Doubts and fears about where I stood with God became a constant source of anxiety. I learned that gluttony was a sin, and the Bible classifies people who eat excessively with drunkards, fornicators, liars, murderers, and evil brutes. It was implied that my obesity was an act of disobedience and that my standing with God might be in question.

The more I listened to the preacher's sermons, the more I felt I was listening to dad. The preacher's messages always included judgment of the evil godless people outside the church, and even included those who were in churches less pure and holy as ours. It was like hearing dad sitting at the head of the dinner table, criticising our neighbours and any person in our community who were on the wrong side of one of his many prejudices.

The dynamics of this congregation were too much like the dysfunction of my family. I was shamed at home and shamed at church. I fell short of dad and mum's approval, and I fell short of God's approval. I was not worthy of earthly love or divine love. Most of my life people had rejected me because I was obese, now it was clear that God hated fat people too.

People at church were generally friendly and smiled at me, but beneath the surface they were no different from anyone else. Instead of empathy and understanding, they quoted bible verses to me, and said they were praying for victory for me to overcome my obesity.

The peace I felt inside me during the worship times of singing, was quickly struck down when the music stopped. The lyrics to one of the many hymns sung in church are:

"Immortal love, forever full,
Forever flowing free,
Forever shared, forever whole,
A never ebbing sea."

But I did not find this full, free, and whole love anywhere else at this church. Instead, this so-called "love" was uncertain, conditional, manipulative, unforgiving, demanding, and something to be earned. The combination of this love and shame was toxic, but it was familiar.

As my involvement continued, my depression worsened. I shared with a church leader about my traumatic past, the damage it had done, and my struggle with my weight and rejection. I was told it was time to stop blaming my past because, "The old is gone and the new has come". This meant I was to forgive and forget my past and pray with faith for God's healing power. But try as I might, I could not leave my past behind. I prayed to God to help me let go, but the healing never came. I was told that "faith moves mountains" and "nothing is impossible with God". It was clear that there was only me to blame. I didn't have enough faith, I didn't trust God, and I was choosing to live in "disobedience". The problem was obviously not God, it was me. It was a story I was painfully all too familiar with.

I knew that seeking professional therapy or a support group would further prove my lack of faith and trust in God. Psychology was on the list of carnal and ungodly things that Satan used to deceive and lure people away from God. The only answer was to persist in prayer.

But the stories I read about Jesus were beautiful. From what I could see, Jesus was not an overly religious person who followed rules, rituals and tradition. He was not ashamed of my humanity. He spoke his mind, partied with the sinners of his day, wept in the face of suffering, embraced vulnerability, expressed anger, and took the side of those that were written off by the religious establishment.

Jesus would not have minded my raw personality and foul language, and there are biblical accounts of him using a few choice words himself. The stories I was most drawn to were of Jesus expressing gentleness, compassion, understanding, and love to those who were hurting.

His message was love. He spoke of God as an approachable and loving father. This was in contrast to my earthly dad, and the God I learned at church who sat upon His throne in heaven, looking down at me judging me for my weight.

Jesus taught that the distinguishing characteristic of knowing God was love—the love of oneself and the love of others. He said the only person I needed to be, in order to gain entrance into God's kingdom of love and grace, was me.

Although I should have run from the church, I didn't. As lethal as it was, it fit the story I had learned about myself. Jenny Marshall was defective, undeserving of love, a problem to others, should be grateful for any crumb of kindness she might receive.

This was how dad saw me. This was how mum saw me. This was how my classmates saw me. This was how my employers and co-workers saw me. This was how church members saw me. This was how the pastor saw me. This was how the masses saw me.

This was how God saw me.

This was how I saw myself.

How could all of us be wrong?

Chapter Twelve
Somebody Loves Me

When you are well over 500 pounds, any kind of significant movement can be strenuous and risky, including walking, lifting, bending over, sitting down, standing up, and climbing stairs. The impact of my obesity was especially felt in pressure placed on my hip and knee joints.

One day I was walking down a rather steep slope and my left foot slipped forward on a strip of small stones. The pressure of my weight sent me tumbling and I injured the tendons around my knee joint. This was the second time I had twisted or pulled that knee in three weeks. I had lost count of the number of times I had done this in my life. Thankfully, I was with my friend Scott who helped me off the ground and offered to drive me home. I was in intense pain and Scott decided on the way back that he would stop at the home of a church member who was a doctor.

Fee was a family doctor. I avoided her like the plague at church because I was too self-conscious about my weight to engage with her. Fee was slim, attractive, intelligent, successful, and carried all the status and recognition of a medical doctor. And there was me—fat, ugly, unaccomplished, expendable, and a nobody. When we arrived, she took a quick look, instructed me to go home and rest, and she would come by in the evening to check on it.

When Fee arrived, she kneeled on the carpet beside my elevated knee to clean the gravel from my leg. As she dipped gauze in water and gently washed out the gravel, she explained why she was doing it. I had never experienced such gentleness. Her tender touch melted me. I felt calmed inside.

While she tended to my injury, she asked me a few questions about myself and my family background. In a moment of unguarded vulnerability, I spilled out my guts, complete with my family ordeal, childhood sexual abuse, and rejection, loneliness and depression. Staring off in space, I indifferently recounted this story as she worked on my knee. When I glanced down, she was looking straight at me with tears sliding down her cheeks.

Rarely had people related to me with direct, steady eye contact, but Fee was giving me her full, heartfelt, and caring attention. There was compassion in her eyes. In that moment I felt accepted, valued, understood, and loved.

If only for those few moments, something shifted deep inside me. A dormant part of me was stirred, something got through to the very core of my being. It was beautiful. It wasn't an instantaneous change-your-life-forever thing. It was a momentary experience, and then it was gone.

Meanwhile, the next week at church I limped down the aisle to the altar after worship in order to receive prayer for my knee. The eldest deacon, Roger greeted me, and I shared with him my physical injury from the two falls, and my struggle with depression. Lucky for me, Roger had a "word from the Lord". Holding one hand above my head and the other on my shoulder, he said that God revealed to him that He allowed me to fall over twice in three weeks to show me that I had to lose weight. If this was true, God was a little late to the party. It wasn't necessary for me to fall and suffer an injury to know I was overweight. I already knew God was infinite in His wisdom.

I limped back down the aisle to my seat, my heart low. God was my last hope, but even God could not bring Himself to accept or love me. I had always been quite literally the elephant in the room, a public spectacle of mockery and shame. It was no different at church. God was like everyone else, when He looked at me, He saw an oversized body but not my fragile wounded heart.

The church taught me that being fat was a sin. I learned only to hate my body more. Not only was my obesity ugly, it was ungodly. I believed that my body was shameful and an embarrassment to God. I believed that I had wasted the gift of my body, my temple, and could offer nothing of worth. My fatness disqualified me from serving God. It was clear that being godly meant being thin.

The church is supposed to be different than the rest of the world, which is what I was depending on when I began attending. But in a culture that is obsessed with being thin, the church is no different.

Christian diet literature and faith-based weight loss is a booming multi-million-dollar industry, guaranteeing the promised land of thinness. Not losing weight is believed to be a failure of discipline and of obedience. Too often, the Christian approach to weight loss is an entanglement of fear-based theology, pseudo-science, and pastoral counselling.

My hopes for finding God's love and an accepting and supportive church community, collapsed into disillusionment. Later in the week Fee called to check how I was doing. To which I responded, "What, physically, mentally or emotionally?!" I felt physically exhausted, mentally wasted, and emotionally empty.

Sensing my despair, she said, "I thought as much." That evening she came to visit.

Looking back now, if it's true that "God works in mysterious ways", then I figure that I was guided toward this church, not to find belonging but to find Fee. She and I were slowly becoming friends, and I was touched by her acceptance, empathy and understanding. I could not seem to find love at church but found it in Fee.

I shared with her more and more about my traumatic childhood and youth, the broken relationships with dad and mum, and the years of rejection and bullying I suffered throughout my school years and in the workplace. I was honest about my food addiction, and the shame, fear, depression, and self-hatred that ravaged my life. As a medical doctor, Fee understood the factors that contributed to and caused morbid obesity. She did not judge me, lecture me, Bible-verse me, or try to save me.

Fee told me that she had struggled with anorexia. She explained its similarities to food-addiction. Both anorexia and overeating came from a hatred of oneself. Instead of denying myself food as a form of self-hatred, I hated myself by overeating. I saw myself as worthless and ugly, and harmed myself with food as punishment.

My pain-filled soul was soothed, and my feelings of shame began lifting as a result. Fee was one of the very few I had met who could see beyond my body. It may have been that as a doctor she viewed bodies in a matter of fact way, that is she did not see my body as the sum of who I was. Fee was interested in knowing and took the time to discover the person I was on the inside. Writer and philosopher, Elbert Hubbard, wrote, "A friend is someone who knows all about you and still loves you." I had never had a friend like this before Fee.

But the gaping hole of shame and self-hatred inside me was too deep and wide for one person or friendship to fill. I saw myself becoming dependent on Fee and desperately clung to her like a life-preserver in a tide of constant emotional suffering. Fee was my lifeline. If I was unable to reach her, I panicked. I often interpreted her mood as meaning that she was done with me. When she gave her attention to others, I felt jealous. I felt childish and beat myself up for it. I had failed as a friend and added this to my long list of failures. It was just like me to ruin a good thing.

Meanwhile at church, it seemed people were suspicious of our friendship. I felt scrutinizing vibes in their glances when I spoke to Fee at Sunday worship services, and other activities and gatherings. I began feeling paranoid, and feared others would warn Fee that I was trouble, and how our close association was unbecoming of an upstanding community and church member. My anxiety about losing Fee intensified, and my insecurities tormented me. I increased what I knew could provide some degree of relief: food, and I sulked everywhere I went.

One Sunday after the service Fee was told that the leadership had "discerned" that I had a "spirit of self-pity", and how I needed to stop my incessant sulking. Fee dutifully visited me to relay the message. In her compassion she interpreted the problem to be one of self-condemnation. We prayed together, and I found some relief in her understanding. Later, I explained to an elder how debilitating my anxiety and depression was, and the elder responded, "What do you want me to say—*poor* Jenny?"

That was the last Sunday I went to the altar for prayer, the last occasion when I would vulnerably share my pain and suffering with others in the church.

Despite the pain of my inner world, rejection at church, and problems at work, Fee was a consistent and steady presence. She had a full life of her own and held her personal boundaries to prevent me from swallowing her whole. But she was mindful of my insecurities and offered plenty of assurances. She did not waver in her friendship and love. The Book of Ruth in the Old Testament tells the story of a deep bond between two women, one in crisis and the other who came to her aid. You might say that I was Naomi who had been crushed by the world, and Fee was Ruth who loyally stood by me.

Irish poet and priest, John O'Donohue, in his well-known book, *Anam Cara*, which means "soul friend" in the Irish language, describes this special bond with these words, "In this love, you are understood as you are without mask or pretension. The superficial and functional lies and half-truths of social acquaintance fall away, you can be as you really are. Love allows understanding to dawn, and understanding is precious. Where you are understood, you are at home. Understanding nourishes belonging. When you really feel understood, you feel free to release yourself into the trust and shelter of the other person's soul."

These words capture the soul connection and sacred friendship I felt with Fee. She saw the real Jenny unmasked. Even the parts I hated most about myself were laid bare before her, and rather than send her packing, she moved toward me with understanding and love. I felt free to release myself into the trust and shelter of her soul. It was beautiful. It was terrifying.

The picture of God I was given at church was an exacting, disapproving, scolding, and unappeasable tyrant, while Fee was the gentleness, empathy, understanding, and love I had longed for.

As our friendship grew, so did the suspicions at church. Deep and loving same-sex friendships are viewed through the lens of homophobia in fundamentalist Christianity. Storm clouds were gathering, and darkness was looming on the horizon of my standing in the church. Fee was a doctor, esteemed pillar of the community, and major tithing member of the church. Then there was me—the fat, unstable, disobedient, wallowing, self-pitying, childish, carnal peon who was sure to lead Fee astray into backsliding and ungodliness.

Oh wait, one more thing.

Now, according to the church, I was an incognito lesbian.

Chapter Thirteen

My Six Hundred Pound Life

It was early afternoon in late autumn. The sun was shining through the narrow window over Fee's dining table and falling near us. We were sitting in her living room, talking. I was on an old lounge chair and she was sitting opposite me. A hurtful conversation with someone at church had sent me spiralling into depression. Tears fell from my eyes and ran down my cheeks as I purged my emotional pain to Fee. As she listened to my story, she looked directly at me with her gentle and empathic eyes.

Fee wasn't like most people. She looked beyond my weight and connected with the person I was beneath. Most never got past the shock of my weight to relate to the human being behind it. Like every human, I carried within me a world of thoughts, feelings, opinions, interests, and yearnings.

I learned early in life that it was wrong to want or need something. Life had revolved around mum, and the emotional drama of the day. No one had time or interest in my state of mind or emotional well-being. The message from my childhood and youth was that my internal world was trivial, irrelevant, selfish, and childish, and that I did not deserve to express myself or be heard.

But Fee was different. She patiently and empathically heard all that I had to say and seemed to feel all that I was feeling. Being heard by her filled my deep-seated human need for connection and restored in me a sense of worthiness and esteem. By listening, Fee was saying,

"You deserve to be heard. I want to know you. Your thoughts and feelings matter to me."

At first, I felt guilty about using up her time and energy. I was incessantly apologetic. She explained that our conversations were not a chore or a mission from God to save my soul, but that she genuinely valued and cared for me. Fee was emphatic, "I'm not here because I have to be, but because I want to be."

Fee got up and walked over to me and placed her hand on my right forearm. Warm sensations radiated through my body like a balm, soothing the most vulnerable and painful places within me. The care I felt was palpable. It was pure and intense and awakened something within me. It radiated from my heart and saturated every molecule of my being. The sensation was so beautiful that I could not resist it.

In that moment, my body, mind and spirit were possessed by something bigger than myself. I was in ecstasy, pure bliss. Something was happening within me, not from an outside source. This was personal, and transcendent. It was right now, and timeless. It was human, and it was divine.

My trust in Fee had triggered this experience. I had opened myself to a love that was so pure and intense that it changed the core of my being. All I could feel was complete love, and nothing else. There was no room for loneliness, heartache, anger, self-hatred, fear, anxiety, or any emotional pain, only love. This was more real than anything I had ever known. Everything else melted away and I was absorbed into these warm, intimate and pure feelings of love, acceptance and joy. I was amazed and overwhelmed by the experience.

Ernest Hemingway wrote, "The world breaks everyone and afterward many are strong at the broken places." My "broken places" were the fractures through which love entered my life. Acceptance embraced me at my wound of rejection, belonging lifted me out of feelings of abandonment, and the sensations washed clean the toxicity of shame.

This beautiful experience deepened my regular life events. I saw more beauty in my everyday life. Journaling, which was already a daily practice, became easier as I allowed this life-source to flow from my heart to my pen and onto the pages of a notebook. This loving presence became an important factor in healing the emotional pain within me. Over time, I gained wisdom through these pages about myself and my life. In the security of love, I could explore my internal world and gain understanding of the unknown areas of my life. Love belongs to all of us, but often we must lay aside what we learned in church to get to it. At least this was my experience.

Meanwhile at church, the pastors, deacons and Elders, along with their Proverbs 31 wives, were watching Fee and I like hawks. The suspicions of my having a covert lesbian agenda to corrupt Fee had become the gospel truth.

Roger, one of the Elders, met with me about my "clinging" to Fee. He explained she needed proper fellowship with church members, implying that I was deliberately preventing her from relating to bonafide and mature Christians in the church.

I told Fee what was happening, but of course no one addressed the matter with her directly. The church leadership didn't want to bother their mascot. The perfect solution was for me to just go away, never to be heard from again.

At a prayer meeting, the pastor's wife shared her "discernment" with Fee that we had an "unnatural relationship" (holy speak for homosexual) that was displeasing to the Lord and could lead to God's "discipline". Fee was advised to end our relationship immediately without telling me. How's that for Christian "community"?

Fee was shocked. She had not seen our friendship in this light before. Horrified that her care had been so misconstrued, she began relating to me differently at church. The deacons prayed over our seats to "break the relationship in Jesus' name". At a prayer meeting we were directed to not pray together, and we were assigned specific prayer partners. The church hierarchy watched our every action. They even drove past Fee's place to see if I was there.

In my desperation I visited Gwen, the pastor's wife, at home. Believing she was trustworthy, I shared one of my journals with her. When I was finished, she sat back with a smug and disapproving look on her face. She said, "Fee is such a wonderful person. We have always known that she was an excellent candidate for marriage. She has so much in store for her." Gwen went on to explain that Fee was such a loving, giving and beautiful person, and God wanted what was best for her, and that I was in danger of jeopardizing this.

Hurt and angry, I said, "Tell me Gwen, am I any value to the body of Christ?" She responded, "Jenny! Watch your thoughts!"

Soon after, I heard that she had brought the topic up at a prayer meeting that I had not attended. The conclusion was that Fee and I were in a lesbian relationship, because I had deceitfully lured her into it and infected her with my sinful lesbian ways. The church leadership increased their efforts to separate us, and it became the #1 topic of "prayer" (read gossip) in the church.

I was reminded that the Bible says there must be "no appearance of evil". Two females spending time together and touching did not look good, and we could not tarnish God's reputation. There was pressure for me to cut connection with Fee and others in the church. It was fine for me to have a relationship with Jesus, just not anyone else.

I was shattered. Roger told another church member that I was "the most unstable person to ever enter the church." Every Sunday was like being in a fishbowl, filled with sharks. So much for finding the love of God in church!

In my journal I wrote about wanting to drive my car off a cliff or into a wall. I questioned why I was alive and what the point of living was. So, I did what was necessary, I cut myself off from love and to escape the pain, I ate.

And ate.

And ate.

And ate.

My weight spiralled out of control. By the time I reached my early thirties I was nearly 600 pounds. My clothes' size was over 32. I wore bloomers as they were the only underpants which fit over my lower abdomen. Getting out of bed in the morning was a struggle. It was exhausting to walk. I was constantly out of breath, sweated profusely, and infections under the rolls of my skin worsened and were terribly painful.

I knew that my obesity was a life-threatening condition, but my addiction had the upper hand. Just like others with an addiction, I had an intense focus on using a substance, to the point that it took over my life. Changes in my brain's wiring caused my cravings to increase which made my behaviour hard to stop. Over time I had built up a tolerance and needed more and more to experience the same highs. Just like every other addict, I was aware of the problem but was unable to stop it.

My addiction was not cigarettes, alcohol, or heroin, it was food. Food was my only comfort. My meals were large enough to feed two people. I would eat an entire cake in one sitting. I was ashamed of myself, but I could not stop.

Accepting love and facing the emotional aspects of addiction was the key to overcoming my overeating. Like everyone else, I craved for something to satisfy me. My substance of choice was food. Food provided pleasure and escape from my painful present. This was how I attempted to fill the void within me, forget my suffering, and anesthetize my emptiness, disconnection, alienation, and emotional pain. But no chemical substance, and not even food, could satisfy this craving. Wholeness cannot be realised through anything we smoke, inject, drink, or eat.

The church often writes off addiction as a "sin" to be condemned, and which can only be fixed by "getting right with God". This represents the ignorance often found in fundamentalist religion when it comes to addiction.

As human beings, we were made to need and desire bonds. As a child and young girl, I naturally needed a loving, unconditional, and safe bond with mum and dad. In the absence of this, I forged a bond with food to give me relief. I could not bear to be present in my trauma, and food offered an escape.

Love is the only solution to addiction. Love says to an addict, "I love you whether you are addicted or not. I love you whatever state you are in. And If you need me, I will come and sit with you because I love you and I don't want you to be alone or feel alone. You are not alone. You are loved." The opposite of addiction is not abstinence. The opposite of addiction is connection.

For this reason, my relationship with Fee was vital for my journey out of food addiction. She personified this love to me. She provided a healthy and loving bond. She also helped me discover this love within myself and showed me the freedom to accept it.

I am often asked how I lost weight. Obesity is a physical, mental, and emotional problem, and each of these must be addressed. However, I would have never experienced healing and recovery had it not been for love.

It was always love.

Chapter Fourteen

Weight Loss by Exorcism

It had never occurred to me that my problem was a demon. That was until the church I was attending planted the seed in my mind. The logic went like this:

- Satan's mission is to overthrow God.

- Satan's strategy is to turn people against God.

- Satan's method involves luring people into habitual sin.

- My obesity was habitual sin.

- My sin separated me from God.

- Therefore, my obesity had a satanic power to it.

- Satan employs demonic possession when necessary.

This logic did not make sense, but I knew I had to lose weight. After all, I'd been told this all my life. I knew of a minister who specialized in "spiritual warfare" and "demonic deliverance". Unlike stories such as The Exorcist, my bed had never shaken violently, I wasn't speaking in eerie male voices or doing vulgar and lewd things, and never acquired superhuman strength. But I was in a vulnerable and desperate state, so I drove seven hours to meet this pastor, Apostle Ross.

Apostle Ross knew part of my story. He explained that he was one of the "chosen" as described in the New Testament, and how God had bestowed upon him the "spiritual gift" of exorcism, which was the supernatural ability to cast out demons from possessed people. He explained that he also involved a team of "prayer warriors" to assist him in his deliverance ministry. Apostle Ross had met with this prayer team and said that they were "told by God" that the time of deliverance was to be 3:00 pm the afternoon of the next day.

This gave me plenty of time to unravel into panic, fear, and dread. What had I gotten myself into? I contemplated shoving everything back into my bags, throwing them in my backseat, and hightailing it home at 76 miles (120 kilometres) per hour, which was fast for my little Hyundai Coupe with a 600-pound possessed woman behind the wheel!

But I decided against it. There had to be an explanation for this curse of obesity that had plagued me my entire life.

It seemed a little far-fetched that evil spirits were behind my food addiction. But after all, Ross was chosen by God and a crackerjack demonologist, and I had driven seven hours to see him. If it were possible for Apostle Ross to exorcise the spirit of gluttony from my mind and body, that just might be the breakthrough I needed. It was time to face the "demon" inside me.

The clock struck 3:00 the next afternoon.

We met in the church hall, surrounded with religious vestments, sacred vessels like chalices, and candles, icons and crosses. The "prayer warriors" were sitting along a church pew, and there was a chair for me to sit on.

Apostle Ross entered the room with a weighty disposition, holding a cross in his hand. My anxiety arose. He asked for prayers to begin. Some stood and began to pray. Some were humming, others were chanting, and some were singing in strange high-pitched tones. In my mind, this alone should have sent any demon packing.

The atmosphere heightened and after several minutes of prayers and chants, Apostle Ross asked the demons inside of me to come out. He asked rather nicely, but nothing happened. The nice approach got nowhere, and he decided to play hard. "Tell me your names!", he demanded loudly. Not a peep. Apparently, he wasn't operating with a full divine voltage and said, "More power Lord!"

My head was buzzing. I was terrified. The muscles in my neck tensed up, and a cold sensation shuddered down my spine and through my body. My stomach was in knots. The others continued praying with more fervour. I could feel the intensity in the room. Apostle Ross held up his cross and screamed, "Demons, come out of her right now in the name of Jesus!"

Nothing.

"What are you feeling Jenny?", Ross asked.

"I feel like vomiting", I said.

He yelled at me, "That's the demons! Stop holding them in, Jenny! Let them out!"

At first, I sat immobilized in fear. I don't do well with people screaming in my face. But then the intensity of the moment reached a breaking point inside of me. I was angry! I was angry that I agreed to subject myself to something so humiliating; angry that I was morbidly obese and couldn't overcome it; angry at the ways I had been judged and rejected by the church; angry that I had to endure the trauma of my childhood; angry at how I had been ridiculed and bullied throughout my life; angry at the disrespect and discrimination I endured at work. Angry! And in that moment, the floodgates of rage burst wide open, and I let out a scream so deafening that it would have expelled an army of demons inside me.

When it came to an end and the dust of my explosion settled, I looked up and everyone around the room was staring at me like I was Hannibal Lector.

Apostle Ross said with holy confidence, "Praise Jesus! The demon has come out!" He told me that the name of the demon had been revealed to him by God. Still sitting in the chair, he called the prayer warriors to make a circle around me and place their hands on my shoulder for a concluding time of prayer. They offered praise and thanksgiving to God for the demon deliverance. I was exhorted by Apostle Ross to "go and be free."

When it all concluded I had a parting conversation with Apostle Ross. I shared with him about mum's death and how it had taken its toll on me. He replied in a monotone voice, "She's dead Jenny. It's time to get on with your life." Apostle Ross definitely did not have the spiritual gift of mercy in his arsenal.

I was relieved that the ordeal was over, and I had survived this episode of spiritual warfare. All indications were that it was a divine success. The demon that had enslaved me to a food addiction had been cast out. I was free.

About thirty minutes into my drive back home, I was craving something sweet. I had a stash of M&M's in my glove compartment. I quickly polished them off, and decided it was best that I just find a place to get a proper meal. I spotted a roadhouse and decided to stop to buy fuel; pizza sounded good. I ordered a meat lovers pizza with large French fries. After finishing my meal, I wanted something sweet. I ordered a rich, dark chocolate cake. I savoured every bite.

Then, I was seized with guilt. Why was I overeating if I had been exorcised of the demon? If the evil spirit behind my food addiction had been cast out, why was I overeating again? Once again I had failed. Even the casting out of demons had not worked. In desperation I clung to the belief that something had happened in me and eventually this behaviour would change.

Years later, Apostle Ross contacted me. He had found a church in my area that invited him to present his workshop on demonology. He asked if he could stay with me at my home. I had another major lapse in judgement by agreeing for him to stay with me while he was here. He indicated that it would just be him coming, and that he only needed a place to sleep at night because he would be busy all day and evening with his workshop.

On his way here, Ross contacted me to say he had decided to bring his wife Beth with him. He explained that Beth informed him that it was not becoming of a married minister and demonologist to be staying alone with a single woman (even an obese lesbian one like me).

I dutifully drove them to the church each day in my little car. It was not easy squeezing Apostle Ross and his celestial ego into the back of my small two-door car. When he and Beth got back to my place the first evening, they were aloof. Beth said that they were focussed on ministering and would not have a lot of time for me. I had given them my bed and I moved to the spare room, but they showed little appreciation.

The next day, I spoke with them about the progress I was making in my spiritual journey. I was excited to share how I was becoming more open to love and coming to a greater understanding of how the dysfunctional dynamics of my childhood had contributed to my weight problem.

Beth responded, "Well, it's about time you got over it!" Apparently, she didn't have the spiritual gift of mercy either. Instead, they questioned my relationship with Fee. Apostle Ross admonished me by stating that I was too dependent on Fee.

Apostle Ross told me to submit to the authority of my pastor and church—the same pastor and church that judged, condemned and belittled me for my obesity; accused me of being lesbian; attempted to sabotage my closest friendship; convinced me that I was possessed by a demon; and told me that the only one to blame for all my hardships, struggles, and difficulties in life, was me.

Ross continued interrogating me about my relationships in the church. I vulnerably shared my difficulty with initiating new relationships. He responded angrily, "If you are not careful, you will have no church to attend!" He then dragged the conversation into an examination of my personal finances, finding more evidence that I was an irresponsible and unstable person.

He topped it off by lecturing me that I could never be right with God unless I obeyed His command to "honour your father and mother." Never mind that my childhood had been traumatic. I tried to explain the abuse I had endured, but Beth piped in, "The Bible says that a child must honour their parents Jenny!" Their message was clear. I could not have any kind of worthwhile relationship with God if I was rejecting the authority of my father. It was a direct offense to God. A condition of God's acceptance was that I obey dad.

Apostle Ross concluded his admonishments by stating, "A woman should be under a man, Jenny." He insisted that I had to be married, under dad, or the pastor of my church. God's way required that I have a "covering" of authority. So, my options were to place myself under my abusive father, a misogynistic pastor, or use a dating service to find a husband. This was worse than the exorcism!

They eventually left. But their visit was a major setback for me. It was clear to me that I wasn't pure enough to receive God's love, which I believed was free for all of us. Apparently, the path was too narrow for someone as fat as me.

The God of religion was becoming more and more like my dad. Coming out from under my dad's authority was one of the most difficult steps I had taken in my life. Now I was being told that submitting to dad's authority over my life was a condition for a relationship with God.

Confronted with the reality of my situation, I considered the facts. My food addiction and morbid obesity had nothing to do with demon possession. The trauma of my childhood and youth were the conditions that led to my dependency upon food for coping and survival. My family genetics as well as mum's own dysfunctional relationship with food had contributed to my food addiction and obesity. There was going to be no quick-fix, magic, secret, or formula to fix it, not even divine intervention or exorcism.

Coming out of my food addiction and obesity would require me to disentangle a web of physiological, psychological, and emotional issues of which I didn't yet know.

What I did know was that I was morbidly obese, addicted to food, and if I did not change, I would die at a young age. My gut was telling me that the trauma from my childhood had played a role, and the shame from this tormented me. Religion had provided no answer and 'exorcism' was not the answer.

But I knew with certainty that love was the key component to overcoming this. The experiences of love I had through Fee, and the discovery of the same love within myself, was a flicker of hope in the darkness of despair. Somewhere inside me, deeper than my shame, there was a part of me that had slowly opened and received love like a flower opening to the light and warmth of the sun. Despite the feelings of shame that had been programmed into me since birth, I knew in my heart that I was loved.

I was at a crossroads. I had explored religion, attended church and turned to God because of my need to find love. But all I found was rejection, hostility, self-righteousness, and indifference. It was clear to me that this whole fundamental religion thing was a farce, and it was time for me to leave it behind.

My involvement had been bittersweet. It was at a fundamental church that I met Fee, and our relationship had become a significant part of my life and still is today. But I was also deeply wounded by my sojourn through the black and white religion of the fundamentalist church. It took me many years to disentangle myself from toxic religious indoctrination. It's one thing to be rejected by my parents, classmates and peers, and employers and colleagues, but it's a whole other thing to feel that I had failed and been rejected by God.

The dynamics at church mirrored my dysfunctional childhood home. As I did with my dad, I exhausted myself trying to please an angry God and feeling like a complete failure. I could never be good enough for either my earthly or heavenly father, and lived in a constant cycle of guilt, repentance, fear, and shame. At church, like home, my thoughts and feelings were abruptly dismissed, and I was taught not to trust them. The misogynistic, authoritarian, controlling and abusive church leadership took a page from the family system I grew up in. Perhaps most detrimentally, my church experience shattered my faith. Any trust, hope, or belief I might have had in God or myself was destroyed.

I had turned to religion in search of love and came up empty handed. But I knew I could not give up on love, even if I had given up on the God of the fundamentalist church.

Chapter Fifteen

What's Love Got to Do With It?

Whenever I returned home to see dad and the farm, it took over two weeks to recover after leaving. Going home was like entering the twilight zone, traveling back in time to the misery of my childhood and youth. Though I was now on my own, held a job, and living independently, dad refused to acknowledge that I was an adult, and related to me in the same dismissive and humiliating ways that he did when I was a young girl.

Each time I visited dad I was deluded into thinking that somehow, he would treat me with respect, and finally give me the fatherly approval and love I had always longed for. Each time I left with the old wound of his rejection freshly ripped open.

The drive from the farm back to my place was three hours, which gave me plenty of time to torture myself over the interactions with dad and my siblings during the visit. Dad's voice thundered in my head with a list of my failings. Always the bad daughter who could never do enough. The last and least child. The fat and worthless one. I would sit behind the steering wheel and drive mile after mile in tears. For the next several days I would be in zombie mode with a monstrous psychological hangover. It would take at least two weeks for the heaviness to completely lift and to come back to myself. Such was the impact the relationship had on my life.

About the time I passed the nearby airport, five minutes from my flat, my mind had shifted away from the memories of my past to the reality of my present life. My spirits had lifted when the airport came into full view, reminding me of Fee and our friendship, and the trips we had taken together.

Unable to give myself love and compassion, I had depended upon Fee for these. It was a huge step to be openly vulnerable with her, to receive what she freely offered. But I assumed that this said everything about her and nothing about me. In my mind, Fee was special because she was able to relate to me in these ways. After all, I didn't deserve it, at least that's the story I had learned from the earliest age. Fee also helped me discover that I could have positive feelings about myself without guilt and shame.

These simple discoveries were the most important for me. I had always depended on something outside myself for my happiness and wellbeing. I imagined that the approval and love of dad and mum would deliver this. Being alone was frightening as I lacked the skills to relate to myself in a loving way.

Through fundamentalist religion I learned that the holy life was granted to the deserving by a God in the sky. But I was never good enough to qualify for this God's love and favour.

For a season I desperately clung to Fee. Whereas my relationships with mum, dad, food, and religion produced hurt and shame, Fee was a stream of unconditional love. Once I learned that Fee's love was trustworthy, I was able to relax into it, and my clingy and desperate feelings began to subside. The fact that she did not allow the church's false accusations to sabotage our friendship, increased my confidence in it.

Through this, I learned to trust myself. Then I could accept that the love I felt when we were together was with me always. That is, I carried it with me and my interaction with Fee amplified what was there already.

My life was saved by love. Coming out of obesity could never save the person I was within, only my body. My greatest personal achievement has always been to remove barriers I had built inside myself to love. In the absence of love, is shame and fear, hence these were central to my food-addiction, obesity and psychological suffering. The foundation of wholeness is loving ourselves. Love is what heals our wounds and brokenness and frees us from the toxic beliefs we learned or created about ourselves. There is nothing that cannot be transformed by love.

It's unfortunate that I never got this message in the church that I attended. Love is the highest expression of any true philosophy, religion, and spirituality. The most profound scripture in the Bible is, "God is Love." God's love does not turn off and on based on our performance. In every moment, we are held in God's love because love is what God is. Love is just another name for God. Religion indoctrinated me with the lie that God's love has conditions which must be met. It took me many years to disentangle myself from this toxic belief and learn to trust and relax into God's unconditional love.

So, if the source of love is within me and God is love, then God is within me. If I was made in the "image of God" and God is love, then I was made in the image of love. Most of my life I had been preoccupied with myself as a fat body, never realizing that love was at the core of my being. It had never dawned on me that I could love myself, and that in doing so was to experience the love of God. At this place of love, God and I were one.

This had many amazing implications. Even though dad's inability to love me was hurtful, it didn't deprive me of love. When mum died, love didn't die with her. When I walked out on the god of religion, I was not leaving any possibility of love behind. If Fee moved away it would not shut-off love to me. My greatest desire in life was to have an abundant supply of love within me at every moment, and now I knew I had this.

As I made these discoveries, I gained greater understanding about my life and my struggle with food-addiction and obesity. I had become addicted to food at an early age because I did not experience true love. This food addiction and my genetics led me to morbid obesity which made me a victim of bullying, discrimination, and self-hatred; this led me back to eating for comfort. Love was the only answer to this; it healed me of shame and gave me faith in myself.

The Bible also says, "Nothing is impossible with God", which I translate as "Nothing is impossible with love." If this was true, coming out of my food-addiction and morbid obesity was not impossible with love. Exorcism couldn't do it, but love could.

Chapter Sixteen
Slow Journey Out of Shame

If making fun of fat people made us lose weight, I would never have been fat at school. If humiliation through mocking obese people and anti-fat bias could curb obesity, then we would be close to eliminating it. But despite the disgracing stigma placed on overweight people, obesity is epidemic. Worldwide obesity has more than tripled since 1975. Over 350 million children and adolescents aged 5-19 are obese.

The only thing fat shaming did for me was make me feel ashamed. This shame led to depression, anxiety, low self-esteem, avoidance of exercise, and self-destructive behaviour like overeating. Fat shaming made me sicker and heavier. "Fat shaming" is just a technical term for bullying. Fat shaming has been proven to increase the risk of suicide.

Most of us would become defensive if we were accused of shaming another person for being overweight. Here are some common characteristics of a person who does fat shaming:

Feels superior in comparison to overweight or obese people;

Makes jokes about fat people seen in public or in the media;

Comments on another's body;

Teases friends/family about their weight in an attempt to be "funny";

Allows for family members to make fun of fat people;

Views thinness as an attribute of success, happiness, or self-control;

Critical and judgmental of others. Assumes weight is a lifestyle choice;

Makes assumptions of personal character/morality based on appearance/size;

Views diets as a quick fix and easy solution to weight issues;

Looks down on others who do not adhere to "clean eating".

A review of the research by the American Psychological Association, indicates that doctors are some of the biggest offenders when it comes to making people feel ashamed of their weight. Studies show that the most common source of fat shaming is family members, and after family comes doctors.

This can be in the form of disrespectful treatment, lectures about our weight, and embarrassing comments. Even well-meaning doctors can ruin a patient's experience if the topic is not approached carefully, and possibly inflict long-term damage to our wellbeing. It is not possible to shame or belittle people into changing their behaviours.

One of the biggest limitations to coming out of obesity was my fear of interacting with doctors and other health professionals. We have all been told that obesity is a personal failing that strains our healthcare system.

For over 60 years, researchers have known two things that could have improved, or even saved, millions of lives. The first is that diets do not work. Since 1959, research has shown that nearly all attempts to lose weight fail and that two-thirds of dieters gain back more than they lost.

The second big lesson is that the terms 'weight' and 'health' are not perfect substitutes. Studies have found that anywhere from one-third to three-quarters of people classified as obese are metabolically healthy. They show no signs of elevated blood pressure, insulin resistance or high cholesterol. Meanwhile, about a quarter of non-overweight people are what epidemiologists call "the lean unhealthy." In fact, unfit skinny people are often more likely to get diabetes than fit fat people. Habits, no matter your size, are what really matter.

One of the misconceptions about obesity is that it is about counting calories and carbohydrates, food choices and willpower. And it is assumed that obesity is caused by a lack of self-discipline, whereas anorexia is a method of self-punishment. However, both have the same root, which is shame. Our society is more sympathetic with anorexics than the obese, because we see anorexics as victims and the obese as the cause of their own problem.

Fat people are not stupid or lazy. We know that being overweight isn't good for us. Obesity cannot be explained as simply a breakdown in willpower. There are many factors that contribute to the condition of obesity. Some of those factors are genetic.

Jeffrey M. Friedman is a molecular geneticist. In 1995, he and his colleagues discovered leptin, which is produced by fat tissue and signals the brain when to stop eating. Research by Friedman has shown that genetic mutations which lead to a full or partial loss of leptin are associated with obesity. Friedman and other scientists identified a number of hormones and genes that play a role in appetite and weight.

Having overweight parents classifies children as at-risk for excess weight or obesity later in life. Children from low-income families are also more likely to face obesity than those from higher income families. Each of us has a unique background, experience, and story. Upbringing, family health history, and family income have a huge impact on health.

So, what is "shame"? Shame is the intensely painful feeling or experience of believing that we are flawed and therefore unworthy of love and belonging—something we've experienced, done, or failed to do makes us unworthy of connection. Shame is a core indictment against oneself.

Whereas guilt says, "I did something bad", shame says, "I am bad." Shame is the conclusion about who we are at the most basic level, that we are worthless, unlovable, defective, inadequate, broken, ugly, a problem, undeserving, to blame, unwanted. I internalized these shame-based beliefs about myself early in life.

Due to genetics, I developed into a big-boned and stocky woman, not a dainty and petite one. One of my first memories was being aware that something was wrong and undesirable about me because of my size. But I turned to food to soothe and escape the internal pain I felt at home. I ate my way through my emotional hurt and pain. This led to an addiction to food which developed into childhood obesity, depression, more rejection, bullying, more shame, and more eating. Childhood obesity led to adult obesity, more depression, more rejection, discrimination, more shame, and more eating. That is how I got to become morbidly obese.

The shame-based beliefs I learned as a child became my convictions against myself. After leaving home, the cast of characters from my childhood and youth were no longer around to reject, bully, mock, and abuse me. It was no longer necessary because I could do it to myself without help. My jailer had changed faces; I had become my own jailer in a cell of self-hatred.

Socrates wrote, "The beginning of wisdom is the definition of terms." In other words, we must get our foundations right if we hope to construct something that is stable. The "terms" I had accepted were my shame-based beliefs about how deficient and pathetic I was, doomed to failure, rejection and loneliness, and deserving abuse.

A few years ago, I was told a story of an elderly couple who took morning strolls along the beach. On their walks they often saw a young boy swim in from the end of the jetty. They were amazed at his stamina. One day, they stopped him as he was making his way from the beach. The elderly man said, "That is an awfully long swim to make, lad."

The boy said, "Yes, I do it every day."

"Why?" asked the elderly man.

"Every day, my stepdad walks me out to the end of the pier and drops me into the water. Then I swim all the way back to the beach."

The elderly couple were astonished. "Why do you do that? That's a big swim for a young boy of your age. It's dangerous swimming that far out."

The boy then said, "It's not the swim that's difficult. The hardest bit is getting myself out of the sack first!"

I identify with the young boy in the story who was tossed into the ocean tied in a sack. The hardest part in my struggle was freeing myself from the sack of self-hating and shame-based beliefs. My problem was not my weight, the way I ate, laziness, or lack of motivation and willpower. It was the shame that defined and ruled my life.

The only solution to shame is love, but shame becomes solitary confinement. I isolated myself from others, believing I was bad and unworthy of connection and belonging. Everywhere I turned there was only shame. When I rang home, there was shame. I attended church and went to work, and there was shame. Just walking out my front door meant I was vulnerable to shame from others. But I figured that it didn't matter. After all, I deserved it. Those were my terms and they were the only terms I knew.

Maybe you are also tied up in a sack of shame, trying to stay afloat in the turbulent waters of life. In my experience, during storms it is enough just to stay afloat. Only you know what you have been through in your life, and you are the only one who knows what your life is like now. Each of us has our own unique journey with its challenges, wounds, and scars.

It's okay to celebrate that you are still here. And it's okay to celebrate how far you've come, and to be proud that you're still standing. Be kind to yourself, have compassion on yourself. Remember to acknowledge your triumphs, which may include just getting through today.

You don't have to be perfect. It is okay not to pressure yourself. It's okay to rest. There is no hidden rule that you must constantly achieve, or that you should please others.

I'm giving you permission to just be where you are and who you are right now. To simply be 'you,' however messy that might seem to you in this moment. Whatever your unanswered questions, fears, disappointments, and wounds, they are a part of you right now. We all have them.

I give you permission to be okay with yourself, as you are today. I give you permission to accept yourself, be patient with yourself, and have compassion on yourself. Permission to stop judging yourself, berating yourself, hating yourself, and finding ways that you tell yourself you are flawed, deficient, inadequate, and don't measure up.

We all want to be more whole and freer. But it's okay not to be whole and free, too. You have permission to like yourself... and to love the 'you' that 'you' are right now.

You are deserving of love, acceptance, and belonging just the way you are. You are deserving of your own acceptance, compassion, and love. There are no conditions you must meet to earn love, acceptance, and belonging.

Rather than punishing yourself about how far you still have to go, acknowledge how far you've already come. I give you permission to be okay with yourself ... all of you ... as you are today. Lay aside your guilt, shame and self-condemnation.

Stop judging and condemning yourself. Question the attitudes and actions that sabotage your happiness and wellbeing. Face them, and challenge them, not to make yourself more lovable, but as an act of love toward yourself because of you are worth the effort. Our greatest achievement in life is to become a person of compassion both for ourselves and others.

Why am I telling you these things? Because I wish I had heard this before.

Chapter Seventeen

Anam Cara

My shame about my weight kept me from loving myself. I believed I was innately bad. This fuelled my self-hatred which in turn fuelled self-rejection. It had never occurred to me that I could love myself, or give myself compassion, understanding, or gentleness. It had never occurred to me that the source of love was within me. I was so unlovable that even God could not bring Himself to love me, even though He was supposed to love everyone.

My belief was that I did not deserve love, which meant I would never find love in a human relationship. To disprove this, I had to be open to love from others. But with all the hurt and rejection I had experienced, I was not willing to take that risk.

A definition of insanity is doing the same thing over and over again and expecting a different result. My own parents, siblings, classmates, teachers, church leaders, employers, co-workers, and many others had rejected me. So, to my mind it was logical that no one else could love me. And even if they did, I would be suspicious of their motives.

This was how I viewed my world.

It was Easter weekend and I had taken Fee to the airport to catch a small plane to a nearby city for a medical conference. She was going to be away a few days, and I felt scared about it. If anything happened to her, I believed it would be the end of me. I desperately needed Fee to be physically present or close, so that I could see that our friendship was real. I certainly couldn't feel that it was real, I was too hurt inside for that. I was still unsure of her love, despite all that she had done for me. I feared her abandonment, so I was afraid of her going away.

When it was time for her to board the plane, I gave her a hug. Not wanting to let go I said, "I think I want to live now." As we drew back, I noticed tears in her eyes. They seemed to be both of relief and pain. "Why are you crying?", I asked. She said, "Because I had wondered what my life would be like without you."

The amount of weight I was carrying was life-threatening, and if I did not do something my life would end early. I was in my mid-thirties and morbidly obese. If I did not change my lifestyle before forty, it was likely that the impact on my health would be irreversible. However, I could not see the point in losing weight as I could see no value in myself.

That is, until Fee had said, "Because I had wondered what my life would be like without you."

At that moment in time, the world stood still for me. Nothing else mattered but those words and how I felt about them. To this day, those few words mark the most significant shift in my heart. This moment was a line in the sand and my life was about to change.

Although I had experienced genuine love through Fee and on my own, I believed it was because she and God were loving me, even though I didn't deserve it. I had always told myself that Fee's interest and care for me was because she was simply a caring person, someone special, a saintly woman, a Mother Teresa type. She cared for everyone. I figured it was her devotion to God, but in my case, it was more like martyrdom.

Those were my self-sabotaging beliefs—anyone who showed interest and cared about me was doing so for some ulterior motive. I could never be worthy of it. It was not possible that I could naturally bring out feelings of affection, care, and interest in another human being.

Looking back, I realize how wrong that was. I denied Fee her right to love me. I projected my shame, self-hatred, and past hurt onto her. Although I had no reason for doing this, I distorted her motivations and insisted that she was no different from anyone else who rejected me. She could not love me; it had to be her devotion to God. My resistance to love was like a thick steel wall.

Perhaps the most tragic consequence of my childhood was not that mum and dad failed to provide the love I needed—it was that the shame I felt about this caused me to seal myself off from love entirely. The one thing I knew—in the pit of my stomach, from the crown of my head to the soles of my feet and deep in my empty chest—was that I would never be truly loved. Looking back, I can see that I had no idea what true love was.

But Fee's words challenged the story I believed. They cut through to my heart, through all my layers of self-protection. My life had been built upon the belief that I was an unwanted intrusion into the world and that my existence only caused misery for others. When it was time to die, no one would notice. I sometimes wondered what the point was and considered taking my own life. I doubted that anyone would really care.

But I had been caught unaware and confronted by Fee's honesty. I could not deny the depth of feeling in her comment. It was the combination of her tears and the honesty which shook my reality. I was unable to withstand her genuine love and concern. Fee said that she could not imagine life without me, and its gravity was authenticated in her tears. No one had expressed anything like this to me before. Most of my life I felt that I never mattered to anyone and I was easily forgotten, dismissed, and insignificant. But to Fee, I mattered. She would miss me if I died. She would experience pain over the loss of our friendship, perhaps even be devastated.

I heard her.

A light came on within me. I felt a deep pang of love and anguish in my heart. Love because I realised the truth in her words—she loved me. Anguish because I had hurt Fee, not just a little, but a lot. The consistent denial of my weight and unhealthy eating and lifestyle had hurt her. This was something I had never experienced before. It had never occurred to me that my obesity hurt others. Up until that point, it had all been about me, and how the consequence of my life and choices affected myself.

But this was not true, it wasn't just about me. My unhealed wounds, food addiction, and obesity had an impact on others, at least it did to Fee. I was hurting my closest friend and the only person I thought had ever truly loved me. This completely changed the way I thought about my weight. I had believed that my weight was bad because it was shameful, and people were embarrassed by my presence. Now I could see that it mattered because it threatened my life, and that would hurt someone. I was hurting Fee and damaging our relationship by not tackling my physical and psychological condition.

When this had fully sunk in, I realized that I could no longer hold onto my story that I was unlovable. Writing off Fee's expressions of love and care as fake, manipulative, or having some ulterior motive, did not line up with her consistent and steady acceptance and friendship. It was not easy for me to accept that our relationship was not a one-way street, and that I provided something worthwhile to Fee, which she valued and cherished.

Slowly I learned how to trust and rest in my friendship with Fee, and the uniqueness of our bond. Anam Cara is a phrase that refers to the Celtic concept of the "soul friend". The phrase anglicizes the Irish word anamchara, anam meaning "soul" and cara meaning "friend".

John O'Donohue writes:

"In this love, you are understood as you are without mask or pretension. The superficial and functional lies and half-truths of social acquaintance fall away, you can be as you really are. Love allows understanding to dawn, and understanding is precious. Where you are understood, you are at home. Understanding nourishes belonging. When you really feel understood, you feel free to release yourself into the trust and shelter of the other person's soul … This art of love discloses the special and sacred identity of the other person. Love is the only light that can truly read the secret signature of the other person's individuality and soul. Love alone is literate in the world of origin; it can decipher identity and destiny."

He also wrote, "A friend is a loved one who awakens your life in order to free the wild possibilities within you … The one you love, your anam cara, your soul friend, is the truest mirror to reflect your soul. The honesty and clarity of true friendship also brings out the real contour of your spirit."

Fee was my anam cara. We were soul mates. A piece of her was in my heart and a piece of me was in hers. We both felt understood and accepted by the other. Our friendship was pure joy. We could relax with each other. I became less desperate and clingy, and secure and confident in our relationship, which has continued and grown to this day, and will continue till death us do part.

My relationship with Fee and the experience of profound love was vital to my healing. Fee's friendship has been my greatest gift in life. Now I had a reason to live. I felt Fee's pain as if it was mine because I loved her. I wanted to take on my obesity for both of us. Instead of living for connection with food, I began living for true connection.

Chapter Eighteen
I Went For a Walk

"A journey of a thousand miles begins with a single step", so says the famous Chinese proverb.

Fee's love for me gave me motivation to do something about my obesity. I did not want to betray our relationship by jeopardizing my health. My lifestyle had to change, and I made the decision to start walking. So, I took my 600-pound self and I walked.

To this day I walk on a daily basis. That is quite an achievement, considering how difficult my first walks were. I decided for my first walk I would take the local streets in the flat area of town where I lived. Putting on my comfy shoes, I headed out the front door and set off. This was the new Jenny, healthy Jenny!

By the time I had reached the end of my street, which was less than a quarter of a mile, I was exhausted. My feet were too wide for my shoes and they were throbbing. My legs were aching, and I was limping. Pedestrians and drivers stared, taking in this distressing scene.

I made it to one and a quarter miles. Every step was excruciating, blisters had formed, my ankles were sore and swollen, my knees ached, and I couldn't move for the rest of the day.

As discouraging as this was, I was determined not to let this new journey end after just one walk. Day two, day three, and day four were not any easier than day one. Exercise was a shock to my body. Up until that point, I had lived a sedentary life.

There were many contributing factors to my weight problem, inactivity was one of them. Recent studies indicate that under-exercising, rather than overeating, may be at the heart of obesity. Surprisingly, we have dropped the amount of exercise we do in our free time.

It is easy to understand why I did not exercise. As an obese child and adolescent, I was terrified of Physical Education classes, which were a cesspit of shaming and bullying. As an obese adult I wouldn't be caught dead in a gym, at a park, or on a trail exercising. I didn't have the resolve to expose myself to the judgement I would most likely experience from others.

Appearance-driven fitness culture has increased our use of body shaming to drive weight loss. Television programs like "The Biggest Loser" isolate their participants from the people and circumstances which influence their poor lifestyle choices. Participants are supported through a rigid exercise and diet regime which leads to quick weight loss. Not only is this unrealistic, it cannot be replicated or sustained in real life. When the participants return to their familiar lives, most put the weight back on or are larger than when they started the program.

After coming out of morbid obesity, I trained to be a functional medicine coach to help others like myself cultivate a healthy lifestyle beyond fad diets and unsustainable exercise regimes. Having done this largely by myself, I believe that I am in a position to help others who struggle with the same issues.

It took courage to change my life, but this is not how I see myself. Instead, I have always thought I was persistent, determined, stubborn. I tend to stick to something until it is finished. In this case, it worked for my good. By doggedly taking one small step at a time I was able to face my fear bit by bit. With each step I pressed toward the goal I was pursuing. It was easier that way. Exercising itself, even without weight loss, was good for my heart and soul. I was doing something about this weight that had burdened me for so long. This was my first step toward health.

That first walk of one and a quarter miles eventually became a painful walk of one and a half miles, and eventually a painful two miles. Anthony de Mello wrote, "Every painful event contains in itself a seed of growth and liberation." Physically these walks were exhausting, but they were also making me stronger mentally, and physically fitter. Each day as I put one foot in front of the other, my self-confidence and self-respect grew.

Over time I attempted longer walks including hills. The first one was gruelling, as I gasped for breath and frequently stopped as I forced my body up the slope. Every part of my body hurt, and sweat poured down my face, arms, torso, and legs. A few people had concerned looks on their faces as they passed me, some worried I would have a heart attack.

With sports shoes, walking every day was easier. There were unintended consequences of exercising so regularly. The weight pressing on my feet numbed my toes. My feet never recovered. The strain on my lower back was immense with all the weight I carried at the front. I could not stand fully upright. I affectionately called the lower abdominal fat and skinfold "Barry the Belly". Barry stretched from my waist and down my thighs. My legs were huge and rubbed against one another, creating painful rashes between them. I went to a podiatrist who made orthotics for my feet, which forced my knees outward to reduce the rubbing.

Fee was a serious walker and loved doing it. She told me once, "I don't walk because I should. I do it because it brings me joy." I did not share Fee's passion for walking, at least initially. I didn't even like walking to my car. Whoever created the remote control was a genius. If I couldn't find a parking spot right next to the restaurant or shop entrance that I wanted, I'd give up and try later.

But in time I began to find great joy in walking. Fee arranged walks we could do together. We explored many surrounding conservation parks, scenic walks, national parks, and botanic gardens. Each little adventure gave me a new sense of freedom and peace. Fee would carry water and food in her backpack for both of us, so that I did not have to carry more weight.

On holidays we would sometimes plan a trip together to scenic areas in the countryside where we could walk together. Fee had the patience of Job. Still morbidly obese, the muscle soreness, sweating, rashes, and fatigue continued to frustrate me. She was forgiving of my slow pace and delighted that she could share with me the joy she experienced from walking.

The fragrance of eucalyptus and other plants filled me with joy. Bees loaded their legs with pollen to take back to their hives. The sounds of nature, like kookaburras and other native birds, were entrancing. I heard kangaroos thumping as they hopped past us. Walking was liberating. Being in nature was healing, soothing, and restoring. I connected with myself, and it was one of my first experiences of feeling happy and grateful to be alive.

Being in nature was some of the best therapy for me. I was away from the gaze of those who judged me for my weight. John Muir wrote, "And into the forest I go, to lose my mind and find my soul." I found these words to be true. Walking in nature was like a vacation from the muddled mess in my head, and a pathway to another world of peace and serenity deep inside myself. I wasn't high on sugar; it was a euphoria of spirit.

We travelled to Kangaroo Island, a small sanctuary not far from Adelaide in South Australia and stayed for a week in a cabin. Although the cabin was one of five, there was no one else there but us. Fee's RAV4, which I affectionately called "Rory the RAV4" was never the same again after travelling back and forth to the cabin along a corrugated road. I felt bad for him—Rory had dirt in every part of his anatomy. Fee and I did shorter and flatter walks together, and she took longer and more arduous hikes on days when I recovered in the cabin.

Walking is the most natural activity on the planet. Henry David Thoreau wrote "Every walk is a sort of crusade." He described the value of walking to his daily life, "I cannot preserve my health and spirits, unless I spend four hours a day at least—and it is commonly more than that—sauntering through the woods and over the hills and fields, absolutely free from all worldly engagements."

Just 45 minutes of walking each day did wonders for me. Walking taught me a lot about myself. I discovered that I could do more than I thought. All my life I thought I was lazy and inept, but through walking I learned I was strong and capable.

Walking didn't require me to be slim or ultra-fit. It taught me that my body was capable of difficult things and the one I had was just fine. I didn't have to achieve some great feat, do an endurance hike, or a race. Instead, I walked at an easy pace which suited me.

Fee bought me some walking sticks to help with my balance. This gave me the freedom to venture off the beaten track to explore nature. As a child I had been too overweight and unfit to do this. The sticks increased my confidence and mobility, which made it easier to navigate uneven and more rugged terrain with my lack of agility. My wanderlust blossomed. It was freeing, and I became the child I had never been.

Next was a walking jacket and backpack. Fee got me a specifically designed backpack which fitted over my hunched, large back. The jacket was made from a waterproof, breathable fabric, which kept me dry.

We did more difficult walks, including climbing and navigating rocky terrain. I often finished these adventures with swollen ankles, bruises, muscle pain, fatigue, and various rashes. But the sense of achievement of pushing through these more demanding hikes strengthened my belief and confidence in myself.

On my 40th birthday we travelled to Lord Howe Island, a tiny island in the Tasman Sea between Australia and New Zealand. We rented bikes to get around. I rode on an adult trike. The beaches were picturesque with crystal clear water and pristine white sand. When we weren't riding our bikes, we walked. Although only 11km long and 2km wide, Lord Howe is covered with dozens of well-marked walking trails; nearly two thirds of the island is a permanent park reserve. The island is World Heritage-listed, and the choice of walks range from easy strolls at sea level through lush kentia palm and banyan forests, to moderate cliff-top hikes where seabirds can be seen wheeling on the thermals, to the challenging Mt Gower climb—rated as one of the best day treks in the world.

We saw several seabird colonies during our walks. There are 14 seabird species based on Lord Howe Island. The flora of the Island is majestic; there are species of flowering plants ranging from tiny herbs to tall rainforest trees 20 metres tall.

At the end of each day my feet were sore, and legs ached, but it was well worth it. Fee found powders and ointments to prevent and heal infections under my rolls of fat and to soothe my skin. It was the best birthday I had ever had!

In the weeks and months which followed, I continued walking. I walked every day and was disappointed on the rare occasions when I couldn't. I wore out countless pairs of shoes, umbrellas, and hats. No matter the weather, I walked. When it was hot during the day I walked at night. I discovered how much I enjoyed walking in the rain. A few times I got caught in a thunderstorm with lightning bolts streaking through the sky. Some got a little too close for comfort and I feared a strike to my umbrella. Other times I was caught in a downpour without an umbrella or coat. I was saturated.

Walking became increasingly more important to me. I loved it. Instead of denying myself food, I walked. Slowly I replaced my overeating with walking. Through my newfound wanderlust, I learned there was more to enjoy in life than food.

As my stamina and fitness gradually improved, my love for nature sparked an interest in gardening. At first it was exhausting, and the pain from the exertion would last for days. Kneeling was impossible, so I bent down. But bending placed pressure on my back because of the weight of Barry. It also made my legs stiff and sore. My back hurt, my legs hurt, my shoulders hurt, my arms hurt, my feet hurt, my hands hurt, my neck hurt, and my head hurt. If it was a body part, it hurt.

But I was on a roll. Many times, I would garden until I was so exhausted and sore that I could not move. Eventually, I learned to take breaks and work for small periods of time. Like walking, I pushed through the difficulties and challenges to enjoy the fruits of my labour. Working my hands in the soil was soothing and made me happy. The tranquillity of the garden gave me peace. Gardening became meditative for me.

I converted my backyard into a small cottage garden. Fee and a few other friends lent me a hand here and there. We created a fishpond with a half wine barrel. They dug holes for me, and we planted roses and small bushes.

Walking and gardening were good for my physical, emotional, and psychological health. They brought me joy. I had always poured myself into trying to make others happy, and it never seemed to be enough. But making myself happy was much less complicated. True friendship, walking in nature, and creating a small garden in my backyard was all it took.

Chapter Nineteen

Stopping the Train to My Early Death

I t sat on my coffee table, calling me. It seemed to speak to my soul. Just one glance in its direction and my mouth began to salivate. It was a large block of Cadbury Dairy Milk Chocolate, my favourite. Resistance was futile.

I unwrapped the top of the bar, closed my eyes, and took in the aroma of the sweet, milky, and chocolatey block. I broke the first row off, enjoying the sight of its brown, milky texture. As I did so, I salivated more. Each square glistened with the word "Cadbury" etched across it. I broke away the first square and placed it in my mouth. I resisted the urge to chew and quickly devour it, which was my usual method. Instead, I held the chocolate on my tongue, savouring the chocolatey, milky sweetness as it melted in my mouth. The sugar rush of ecstasy went straight to my head.

My intention was to have only one row of the chocolate squares. It wasn't that much, and I knew I could stop anytime I wanted. After finishing the top row, I decided to have one square off the next row. It had been a stressful day. My body was fatigued, both physically, and emotionally. My head was throbbing from the tension in my neck. I just wanted some pleasure to negate the unpleasant feelings of the day. I liked how chocolate made me feel. "It's not like I eat it all the time …" I told myself, " … it's only a few pieces of chocolate."

Caught in the pure delight of the sugary rush and milky bliss, I had a few more squares until I had devoured the entire 12-ounce (350g) block of chocolate. The high was heavenly but then the sugar withdrawal set in. The depression from the binge always lasted longer than the high from the sugar rush. My body would become fatigued. Then I would look for more sugar to pick me up again.

I didn't understand at the time, but I was addicted to sugar. Any recovering alcoholic could identify with the lies I told myself about my addiction—"just one more", "I can stop whenever I want", I'm stressed and want to relax", "It's only a few pieces", "I'm not as bad as ______________."

Excess sugar can be as addictive as drugs and have similar effects on our brain. Too much can lead to addiction. When we eat sugar, our brain produces dopamine in large amounts, giving us short term pleasure. Over time, eating large amounts of sugar changes the function of our body so that we need more to experience the same effect. This is similar to the reaction to heroin and cocaine and is the link between added sugar and addictive behaviour.

With the excess release of dopamine and other messenger molecules, we feel a pleasurable "high" which is followed by withdrawals. The discomfort experienced by the withdrawals drives us back to ingesting more of the substance to relieve the withdrawals. Over time, we need more to have the same affect, so the only way to relieve the withdrawals is to repeat the process in increasing amounts and frequency. This is substance misuse which is the process of addiction.

Despite the negative consequences like weight gain, headaches, and hormonal changes, my cravings for sugar continued and I kept eating it. Every time I ate sweets, cakes, or cookies I reinforced this process, causing my brain to become increasingly hardwired to crave sugar, and at the same time building up a tolerance to it.

Unlike alcohol, sugar is readily available to children. Hence, I developed a sugar addiction early in life. It was a vicious cycle of binging, withdrawal, and cravings. As my body could not use all the sugar I consumed, it stored it as fat. Stored fat impairs the effectiveness of insulin which means our body must make more insulin. When more fat is stored in our body's fat cells, those cells produce more abnormal signals, which then make the metabolism more abnormal.

In her later years, mum experienced many health problems because of her food addiction. She developed diabetes and eventually ulcers on her feet and legs. We worried that she would develop gangrene and require amputation of her toes or feet. Her eyesight became weaker, and she lost feeling to her fingers and feet. Eventually she developed septicaemia, which weakened her heart. Septicaemia is a serious bloodstream infection. The clinical report at the time stated that a piece of infected flesh, most likely from the heart, lodged on the right side of her brain, causing a stroke.

Food was the bond that held mum and me together. Mum reminded me of the enjoyment I experienced from food. We were the perfect enablers for each other. A child with one obese parent has a much greater chance of being obese. When both parents are obese, their children have an even higher risk of becoming obese. Parental obesity more than doubles the risk of adult obesity among both obese and non-obese children.

The food environment created by our parents is vital to the behaviours and attitudes we develop as children about food. Parents expose their children to certain foods, portion sizes, feeding styles, role modelling, physical activity, sedentary behaviour, and the family routines they create. These interactions teach children how to eat, exercise, and cope. So, children are more at risk when their parents experience an eating disorder or suffer from obesity.

As a child and adolescent, I was fuelled by my addiction to food. No amount of fat shaming could change this behaviour, and only led to more eating to anesthetize and escape feelings of self-hatred, rejection, and depression.

Although walking had become a life-changer for me, it did not resolve my sugar addiction. I tried many ways to improve my eating habits, like reducing my sugar intake and eating more protein-rich foods. My plan was to snack on food items like nuts instead of sugar-filled highly processed foods. My theory was that if I could eat food which was more filling that was less addictive, then eventually I could wean myself from overeating.

There are many misleading messages about the food we eat. For example, carbohydrates are not bad. Our brain uses carbohydrates to function. When we move, we need carbohydrates. They are neither good nor evil; they're just fuel.

Mary Bray Pipher said, "Girls developed eating disorders when our culture developed a standard of beauty that they couldn't obtain by being healthy. When unnatural thinness became attractive, girls did unnatural things to be thin."

The weight loss supplement industry is massive. The main reason supplements work for some people is the placebo effect. We fall for the marketing tactics and want the supplements to help us lose weight, so we become more conscious of what we eat.

The diet industry drives many unfounded myths, including:

All large people are in poor health and *must* lose weight in order to improve their health and fitness level.

Everyone can lose weight IF they just follow the proper diet and regular exercise program.

The main reason people regain lost weight is *their* failure to comply with prescribed diets.

Being underweight is *better* than being overweight.

The nutritional costs of fad dieting are harmful. Adhering to a strict diet can mean depriving our body of the nutrients it needs, which does not support good health. Dieting also takes a toll on mental health.

Over the years, I tried a few diets. From experience, dieting is stressful. I was constantly fighting and denying myself what my brain and body wanted. There was no quick fix for me. Changing my food intake was not just about reducing the amount of food, fat, and sugar I ate; I also had to deal with my addiction to sugar. These dynamics tied together with my belief that being fat made me bad was a dangerous combination. I saw my weight as something that I needed to "fix" about myself, and when the diet didn't work, I blamed myself and took it as a personal failure.

There is no one food plan that suits everyone. Each of us has a unique metabolism, nutrition needs, tastes, and food sensitivities. For example, beans made me bloated, and nuts and avocados were better proteins for me. Cow's milk contains lactose, which caused me stomach pains. I used lactose-free milk as an alternative. I tried artificial sweeteners, but they only increased my desire for sugar, and the unhealthy chemicals contained in these created further health risks.

Eventually I settled on a low Glycaemic Index (GI), low-fat, higher-protein diet with reduced sugar. This worked for me as it satisfied my hunger. My eating plan on a good day consisted of:

- muesli, protein powder, crushed nuts, and lactose-free milk for breakfast

- fish, tomatoes, celery, raw carrots, cheese and bread for lunch

- lean meat and cooked vegetables for dinner

- nuts as a snack between meals

In the end, I discovered that what matters most when it comes to exercise and eating is developing healthy habits. This not only applies to fitness and food, but also to areas such as sleep, stress-reduction, self-care, and mental health.

Changing my way of eating made me feel better about myself and improved my overall health, but it did not solve my addiction to sugary comfort food. I regularly fell off the wagon with a box of chocolates or a bag of potato crisps.

It was time to face the fact that my sugar addiction and eating issues were not about what I was eating but why I was eating it. High sugar foods were the staple of my childhood diet. I associated these foods with love because they were the primary bond between myself and mum.

I learned that the sugar rush of junk food was the happy place that lifted me out of the feelings of shame, rejection, anxiety, and fear which consumed my life. I didn't eat because I was hungry. I ate to feel better. The purpose of food for me was not to satisfy my physical hunger, but to appease my emotional hunger.

Emotional hunger can't be filled with food. Eating felt good in the moment, but the feelings that triggered the eating were still there. In fact, I often felt worse after I had eaten than I did before, because of guilt. I would berate myself for what I had devoured and for my lack of willpower.

Emotional hunger was a powerful driver for my food addiction. It led to mindless eating and feelings of powerlessness. I knew that filling myself with food did not satisfy this hunger. My hunger was not driven by my stomach but by my soul. Exercise and food are vital for good health, but I needed to do more than this. I had to dig deeper to get off this well-worn track which was leading me toward an early death.

Over time, I endeavoured to understand myself. Learning healthier ways to deal with my emotions, gave me more control of my weight and increased my power over both food and my feelings.

Chapter Twenty

The Kitchen Is Not Paradise

After an emotionally exhausting day at work I walked into my empty flat, replaying in my head all my failures of the day. Once again, my supervisor had angrily accused me of being slow and unmotivated. He often buried me under a pile of work which was impossible to complete on time. I wasn't a mind reader, so I had no idea which jobs he wanted prioritized. Just like many others, he disliked fat people and saw my obesity as personal failure on my part.

When I walked through the front door, the emptiness of my flat felt heavy and despairing. It was the same feeling when I put my feet on the floor each morning. I woke up alone. Ate breakfast alone. Came home after work alone. Ate dinner alone. Watched television alone. Went to bed alone. The emptiness of my flat was suffocating, and a reminder that I deserved this fate to be alone.

Most women my age had married, sometimes more than once, or were in a romantic relationship. Where I came from, this is what normal women did. But I was not normal. I was fat. I had never even dated.

Mum explained to me early in life that men don't like to date or marry obese women, that I'd always be single and need a career to support myself. My obesity and sexual abuse made me ashamed of my body. I was awkward socially and had no self-confidence. I was terrified of sex, and mistrusted men. This wasn't the right formula for attracting Mr. Right. I had to lose weight and be thin to find love.

There were days when living by myself felt like solitary confinement. I had no one with whom to share my feelings or experiences of the day. Being home alone often triggered fear and anxiety.

Loneliness was one of my greatest wounds. It was the setting of my life as an obese person. My loneliness felt like I was hungry when everyone around me was enjoying a feast. But it was not just hunger, it was psychological malnutrition, the lack of something I needed to survive. Psychologist, Abraham Maslow created the Hierarchy of Needs as a way of describing the needs of all human beings. After food, water, shelter, and safety, Maslow said that we needed our psychological needs met, psychological needs such as belonging, love, and intimate relationships. Loneliness is unnatural; we were made to be in relationship, not isolation.

Long-term feelings of loneliness can affect our health. For example, chronic loneliness can lead to stress and anxiety which causes the body to release cortisol. Over time, this can lead to problems such as inflammation, excess weight gain, insulin resistance, and problems concentrating.

Loneliness was a dark place where I believed that my life mattered to no one. I felt rejected, unwanted, and unloved. For me, loneliness meant suffering alone. But it is more than being physically alone, I felt alone even when I was with others.

Despite my struggle with living alone, I had one happy place: the kitchen. On that evening, I came home and was in self-hate mode. My depression worsened as I analysed what had happened during the day, finding fault in everything I did. I knew how to relieve this pain, at least temporarily. In the kitchen was a jar of peanut butter and a fresh loaf of white bread.

I took the jar from the cupboard and spread a thick layer on a soft, white piece of fluffy bread, and wolfed it down. I ate the entire slice in two bites. The rich, salty, sweet paste and soft, white bread was euphoric, and I felt a little less alone. Some of the paste stuck in my throat making it difficult to swallow. After filling a large cup with milk, I drank half of it in a single gulp. It was painful as the milk forced the lump of peanut butter down. When the obstruction had gone, I decided there was room for more and did it all over again.

Beginning as a young child I learned that food was the solution to my loneliness. It was the closest thing I knew to love. Mum gave me food and when she was not present, this is what I used. This was our bond. Our closeness was based on emotional eating and food addiction. When mum was eating, she seemed happy. When she was not around, I could eat and feel she was with me.

Other times, love had to be earned. When I told mum I loved her, she would often respond with, "You don't tell people you love them, you DO things for them!" The problem was that I could never do enough or didn't do the right things. I was five years younger than my next sibling, which meant they were always able to perform better than me.

Mum expected loyalty to her if I was to obtain her love. Succeeding was an impossibility. She was always in one crisis or feud with dad after another. The weight of her unhappiness was heavy and wearying. I was afraid of displeasing mum. Her punishment was indifference.

It wasn't until I had left home that my journey of discovering true connection and intimacy started. As devastating as mum's death was, it enabled me to free myself from her control and my fear of her abandonment. Fee's love and friendship was crucial in healing my relationship with myself.

It took me years to develop a relationship with myself. As I found the courage to explore what I needed and wanted, and my wounds and beliefs about myself, I grew in self-awareness. Self-acceptance did not come easily; it took a long time before I could look at myself without judgment or shame. I learned to give myself compassion when I felt inadequate, experienced setbacks, or failure. Building self-trust, self-confidence, and self-reliance was a daily battle.

My greatest successes had nothing to do with a number on a scale, or my waist size. My true triumphs were letting go of shame, loving myself, and living with self-respect.

What I most needed could not be served up on a plate. What I found in the kitchen could not heal my wounds. The right place was deep inside of myself where the true me could be found, waiting to be heard. I was the only one who could hear me at this depth, and it must be with love.

Chapter Twenty-One

Fat Women Can't Be Feminine

Like all the farmers in the district, dad had petrol tanks for the vehicles on the farm. The large, round tanks were laid on their side making it easy for us to climb them. At one end of the tank was a fuel pump used to fill the vehicles and at the other end was a tall pipe to release pressure. In the middle of the tank was a plug where it was refilled. This was a perfect play horse.

As a little girl, I would copy my older sister and climb them. We imagined we were riding racehorses, the fuel pump being the head. Our legs straddled the tank, and we would kick our heels and pretend to be racing to the finish line.

On one particular day I played alone on the tanks. It was hard pulling my chubby little body to the top without someone older to help. But with all my effort I managed to hoist myself up the tank and assumed my riding position. I kicked and coaxed the play horse to victory in the Melbourne Cup, Australia's most famous annual thoroughbred horse race.

When it was time to dismount the tank, I thought it would be fun to first climb the petrol tank beside it. They were situated close together and I thought it would be easy to go from one to the other. As I was lifting my leg over the fuel pump, I lost my grip and slid down the side between the two tanks and got stuck. There was nothing I could reach to pull myself out, and the more I wiggled the more I became hopelessly wedged between the tanks.

Lodged between the tanks, it was becoming increasingly painful. Nobody knew I had gone out to play, and I feared it would be hours before anyone knew I was missing or even cared. My frightened mind went wild as I imagined being stuck all night or even days, or maybe forever between the two tanks. Panic set in and I began to scream for help.

A few minutes of wailing passed when I saw dad walk out of his workshop nearby. I could tell he was angry. I had interrupted his work. With some effort, he pulled me out from between the tanks. He indignantly shook his cigarette at me and bellowed, "You shouldn't be playing on these. You are not like other kids. You are too fat!"

I discovered as I got older that I was too fat for many things. Too fat to ride a bike, too fat for school desks, too fat for bus seats, too fat to play sports, too fat to swim, too fat to buy clothes in normal stores, too fat to wear jewellery, too fat to have a boyfriend, too fat to get in and out of cars, too fat for airline seats, too fat for restaurant booths, too fat for bathtubs, too fat for movie theatre seats.

Mum pumped shame into me about my size and appearance from an early age:

"You're too heavy to sit on me."

"Look how much bigger you are than the other kids."

"You are too slow."

"You embarrass me."

"You stink."

"You'll never be attractive."

"No man will ever want you."

During my teen years mum and dad's marriage deteriorated. I was mum's surrogate husband. She would pour out her emotional pain to me, and she would seek me out for hugs and physical affection. Although our relationship was not sexual, mum was receiving from me the emotional and physical closeness she would have had with my dad in a healthy marriage. I was anxious and conflicted about the kind of relationship I had with mum. I enjoyed her attention and craved her touch, but somehow it seemed wrong.

Mum and I were enmeshed together in so many dysfunctional ways. There were no boundaries between us. I didn't know where I ended, and she began. I found the weight of her misery overwhelming, and I often felt responsible. I was constantly worrying about mum's problems. We had a one-sided relationship—I was her emotional caretaker and she turned to me to comfort her pain and meet her needs, while my hurts and needs were ignored. When mum was happy, I felt balanced, stable. But when she was indifferent or emotionally withdrawn, I felt like a ship without a mooring. I was terrified of her abandoning me and jumped at her command.

Puberty was a confusing and damaging season of my early life. Like other mothers of her era, mum never talked with me about puberty or what to expect. When she started noticing changes in my body, she assumed it was due to hormonal changes from weight gain.

Mum told me that I couldn't be attractive because I was too fat. She had no compassion when I started menstruating, which was frightening. At first, I thought one of my many ulcers had burst. I went to the kitchen where she was preparing dinner to show her the blood. She angrily yelled that she did not know what do to about it. "Stop your whining!"

One thing was clear to me: my body was bad and wrong, and my only hope was to not be fat. If I wasn't fat my body would be good. If I wasn't fat, I would be happy. If I wasn't fat others would accept me. If I wasn't fat, I could earn the love and attention of others. If I wasn't fat mum could be a mother to me. If I wasn't fat dad would be proud of me. I would do anything to lose weight. The only problem is, I could not stop eating.

As I stumbled into adolescence, I could not see myself as a young woman, let alone an attractive one. The awakening of sexual desires scared me and made me feel dirty. I never had a conversation about sex with my parents, but I did overhear my dad telling one of my older sisters that if he ever found one of them having sex, he would disown them. Mum told me that men did not find fat women attractive.

I hated being female. I felt ugly. Femininity was a characteristic of dainty and petite girls; not burly brutes like me. Even without my obesity, my natural stature was big-boned and stocky. Being fat was adding insult to misery. Even my hands were fat. However, during my adolescent years I discovered that the fatter I was, the more unattractive I was to boys, which kept them at a safe distance. They petrified me. My obesity isolated me from others but was also a useful means of self-protection. On some days my fat was like a shield, protecting me. On other days it was like a blanket, holding me close and comforting me.

I expected that my future would not include men. Dad was the first male in my life. Boys ridiculed and bullied me in school. As a child, male doctors and dentists had been judgmental and harsh. When I entered the workforce, I was a victim of discrimination at the hands of men. The religious world I entered was patriarchal, misogynistic and sexist. Even the god of religion was a man and he wasn't particularly fond of me. The common denominator among these was fat-shaming and rejection.

I had many reasons to eat. At an early age, overeating affected my mental health and permanently damaged my body. I developed lipodystrophy: an uneven distribution in fat cells on my legs which led to one being bigger than the other. Obesity led to my developing knock knees, causing them to shift inward until they touched and pushed my feet out. My heaviness caused bad posture. It bent my spine, causing me to walk hunched over so that I looked like Quasimodo in *The Hunchback of Notre Dame*.

Obesity cost me many things in life. It cost me my physical and mental health. It robbed me of career opportunities and friendships. It was at the heart of my mistrust of men and of a healthy partnership with one. It made me feel like a failed woman. Obesity cost me love as I did not believe I was worthy of it, so I could not accept it when it was offered.

It was difficult to see myself as anything other than a victim until my mid-30s. I had been victimized most of my life. How I had been treated was wrong, and inexcusable; its impact on me was catastrophic. The system is rigged against obese people. Weight discrimination and fat-shaming is a socially acceptable injustice.

But choosing to see myself as someone who was in control of my own life gave me freedom. I came to a point when I realized that even though others may have hurt me, I was the only one who could allow myself to heal. For a long time, I had searched for someone to rescue me, but there was no cavalry coming and no one to save me.

Love was the only answer. I had to make the decision to accept the love I experienced within and from those around me. That meant having the courage to ask for help. It is normal to feel sadness, sorrow and anger about being victimized, and indignation toward those who hurt us. But I had wasted too much emotional energy on these things and needed to redirect it toward my own recovery by focussing on love.

Maybe you have been victimized, abused, and rejected in your own life. I understand and care. If I could, I would reach out and hug you to take your pain away.

Shame has been the most damaging influence in my life. But now I realise that my wounds are avenues into the best and most beautiful part of who I am. In these wounds I experienced love. I want you to know that you're beautiful too. I'm telling you because I don't know if anyone else ever has.

Chapter Twenty-Two
A Doctor Named Cathy

I feared doctors, particularly men. It took me a while to get over the fact that Fee was one. When I first met her, I said, "I wouldn't go into a doctor's office with a 10-foot pole!"

At the time she replied, "Oh, I don't have one of those in my office!" Fee had a gentle and quick wit. She wasn't what I expected.

Mum told me more than once that doctors would not want to see me, that they would judge me for my weight. Mum managed to align my weight with every illness or ailment. Whether it was a sprained ankle, knee, bed wetting, seasonal allergy, or spider bite, it was always because "you are too fat."

Sadly, there are studies that show that obese people are more likely to receive inadequate medical care and be misdiagnosed. The research indicates that it is not uncommon for some doctors to advise weight loss for fat patients instead of referring them for other services, as they assume their weight is the reason for the symptom. Because of this, many obese people avoid doctors.

Experience has taught me that hospital gowns don't fit obese bodies, most blood pressure cuffs are not made for large arms, and most scales have a weight limit. Not all doctors' office chairs are suited for the average weight and are not large enough for people with obesity.

My newfound love for gardening forced me to face my fear of the medical world. While cutting back my rose bushes, I cut myself on a thorn. It was a deep cut, which ran down the outside of my thumb. I bandaged it up and showed Fee the next time I saw her.

She said, "When was your last Tetanus shot?"

My gut knotted up instantly. There was no way I was going to a medical clinic of any sort. I couldn't remember ever having a Tetanus shot after primary school. I told Fee this to which she replied, "You'll need to get it done." This was not what I wanted to hear. I thought of risking Tetanus, or letting my thumb go gangrenous, but this would most certainly land me in hospital.

Fee told me that the local council offered free vaccinations, including Tetanus. I told her I'd first give it a few days and keep me eye on it. She responded by explaining that Tetanus was a serious bacterial infection that releases toxins which can lead to painful muscle paralysis and prevent breathing.

I contacted the local city council for the date of the vaccinations. But I managed to confuse the date for the vaccination and missed out.

What was I going to do?

Perhaps Fee would give me the vaccination herself. But that would still require me going to a clinic. The journey of a thousand miles was going to require another step. It was time for me to pull-up my big girl panties and face the music.

The next day Fee and I were in her car on the way for a walk. I told her that I had messed up the dates for the Tetanus vaccination and would not be able to get one from the local council. There was a long foreboding silence. Then, almost involuntarily, I blurted out, "I'll go to the clinic for the vaccination. While I'm there, I'll get my blood pressure, blood sugar levels, and cholesterol checked."

What had I done? Did I really say that? The car was filled with silence. Maybe Fee didn't hear it. Nope. There was no turning back now.

Tears of relief filled my eyes. I had taken another step in facing the shame that had controlled my life. For a moment I felt a pang of fear, but it quickly evaporated as deep peaceful feelings flooded my inner being. Whenever I took a small step in the direction of caring about myself or took an action that improved my health and wellbeing, I felt love, whole, light in spirit, and weightless inside. Saying no to fear and shame and saying yes to love was liberating.

Wiping her own tears away from her eyes, Fee said softly, "I was hoping you would do this. I didn't want to nag or pressure you, but I prayed you would." Fee and I were like family, sisters. She believed that we were too close for her to be objective when it came to my health and medical decisions. We both knew it was not healthy for her to be my doctor.

I asked Fee if she would see me for the first doctor visit and check-up. When the day came, I was filled with apprehension. What if I had diabetes like mum? What if my blood pressure was incredibly high and it could not be controlled? What if I had liver or kidney disease?

When I entered the clinic, I waited with the other patients. Eventually, Fee waved me into her office. Her understanding and empathy helped calm my nerves. We chit chatted for a few minutes, giving me time to relax. She brought out the large blood pressure cuff which would fit around my arm. My blood pressure was high, but she said it was at a level that could be managed with medication. Relief filled me.

She also organized blood tests. I feared what they might reveal. Mum had diabetes at 36, when she was pregnant with me, and suffered with it for the rest of her life. I was far more overweight than mum. It was a distressing few days waiting on the test results, but when they came back, they were all good. It amazed me that I had reached my mid-thirties without succumbing to diabetes. I had been well over 250 pounds since childhood.

Fee then arranged for me to see one of her colleagues, named Cathy. I was uneasy, not knowing what to expect. She was a woman, but the only doctor I had ever felt comfortable with before that day was Fee. What if my doctor was like mum had always said? What if I received a humiliating lecture about how I have to lose weight?

My anxiety rose as I sat in the waiting room of the clinic for Cathy to call me into her office. As an obese woman with great rolls of fat in a doctor's waiting room, I felt like the elephant in the room (no pun intended). Per usual, people went back and forth between staring and trying not to stare.

I began having second thoughts. Maybe this was all just a huge mistake. I contemplated how I might escape the clinic. Walking out the front door was too obvious, one of the receptionists would notice. My only possible option was to claim that I left my phone in the car. As I weighed my getaway options, I heard a voice call out, "Jennifer Marshall."

There Cathy stood—a thin, petite, attractive woman. Honestly! I followed her as she led me back to her office. Yes, I was the Hunchback of Notre Dame following Cinderella down the hallway into the Temple of Doom.

She motioned for me to take a seat, and I sat on a chair beside her desk. I watched as she folded her tiny legs around each other. I couldn't even cross mine! She looked up at me with a warm and caring smile and asked, "Would you prefer to be called, Jennifer or Jenny?" "Jenny", I replied. She continued, "Okay, Jenny. So, how can I help you?"

Her demeanour and question threw me. I expected her to have a condescending tone in dealing with me. Cathy seemed gentle and compassionate. And I could count the number of people on one hand throughout my life who asked me something like, "How can I help you?" She was interested in my needs and concerns. I found Cathy's warmth and genuine attention both assuring and awkward.

In response to her question, I began rattling off a list of things and didn't know where to stop. I told her about my high blood pressure. My family's health history, and my lifelong problem of obesity. How I had struggled to lose weight. I told her about my fear of developing diabetes and dying early.

Cathy let me speak, and she listened. It wasn't patronizing; it was an earnest, genuine, caring, and dignifying kind of listening. She looked over my file and saw my blood pressure and prescribed medication. Cathy explained that my high blood pressure was hereditary and that I should not blame myself. I was surprised to hear this from her. I expected her to blame me for my blood pressure. I had been told that my mum's health issues were entirely related to her weight. Over the next several months, Cathy's words proved true. My weight loss did not improve my blood pressure. When we finished our conversation, she arranged for one of the nurses to give me the Tetanus shot.

Cathy became my usual doctor, and over time we developed a familiarity and connection. It was her accepting, compassionate, and genuine way of relating to me that changed how I thought of doctors. It also increased my willingness to seek and accept the help of the medical community in addressing my morbid obesity.

One afternoon I managed to walk directly into the corner of a cupboard at home. It hurt! A bruise developed on my chest and the next day I noticed a lump on my breast. Cathy wasn't available so Fee recommended I see Todd at the clinic.

"Todd"? Todd was a male …

Then it sunk in a little deeper. "Todd" was going to check my breast! I had never exposed this part of myself to anyone before, let alone a man.

I was a mess that day when I showed up at the clinic. But as it turned out, Dr. Todd was not skinny, young, or pompous. He was on the stocky side, had grey hair, and was meek mannered. He walked me back to his office, where we had a conversation about my health overall and a few issues related to my efforts to lose weight.

Following all of this, he explained what was involved in checking my breasts for lumps, particularly the one I had already found. Seriously? The look on my face must have been priceless.

Dr. Todd said he was going to step out of the room momentarily and asked that I remove my bra and sit on the examining table. I was mortified that he was going to do the breast check with me sitting up. It wasn't just the usual feelings of exposure most women experience but was compounded by all my saggy skin. By this time my underarms were saggy from empty skin. I had lost a lot of weight in my shoulders, face, and breasts, but not so much in the rolls beneath this area. It was as if I had stood beneath a hot lamp and the fat had melted at my shoulders and run down my body. The rolls of fat beneath my breasts were still large.

Horribly embarrassed, I said to Dr. Todd when he re-entered the room, "I'm all saggy-baggy, Dr. Todd, and I've got scars from the ulcers I had when I was a kid." He said, "That's in the past now Jenny. You're doing good." During the examination he could find no additional lumps but referred me for a mammogram for the one lump that he confirmed I had.

A week later I visited the local hospital for the mammogram. I checked in at the front desk and took a seat in the waiting room. I was flicking through a magazine when I heard this delicate voice call my name. Of course, the technologist had to be a young, slim, blonde woman.

In the room, she asked me to undress and put the gown on backwards for the x-ray. There was that horrifically awkward moment when it became clear the gown was not going to fit, exposing my rolls of fat. Seeing the problem, she said, "I hate hospital gowns. I apologize, just do the best you can." Doing the best meant holding the gown across my tummy to hide my rolls.

She kindly asked me to move as close as possible to the glass plates. Getting close was near impossible with my fat rolls and hunched back, but I managed to remain in the most uncomfortable position for long enough to have the mammogram. Noticing my discomfort, she said that there were women bigger than me and not to feel bad about myself. She seemed genuine and I appreciated her attempt to make the best of a discomforting experience. I felt deep compassion for those women who were 'bigger than me'. A few days later I received a call from the clinic. To my relief, the lump was nothing of concern.

For most of my life I have hated my body. Mum frequently pointed out all its problems, which included being big boned, obese, knock kneed, bad postured, and short necked. Dad once told me that I smelled and was not attractive.

My body was judged, mocked, shamed, and bullied by many of my classmates and teachers throughout my years in school as a child and a teenager. In the workplace, I was a victim of discrimination and often found myself being harassed and unfairly treated. At church, my body was my greatest sin and offence to God, and proof of my carnality, and lack of faith and devotion. It was Jenny with the Terrible, Horrible, No Good, Very Bad … Body.

But then a succession of unsuspecting people suddenly started appearing in my life in places I would have never expected. The same fundamentalist church that attempted to deliver me from the demons, turned out to be the link that connected me with Fee. My gardening fiasco that forced me to see a doctor, resulted in my experience of meeting Cathy. In the process I discovered that even a slim blonde and a male doctor can be genuine human beings who are caring, compassionate, kind, and respectful.

Those of us who struggle with obesity are not just bodies in need of medical intervention or someone's research project; we are human beings with hurts, insecurities, and fears, and in need of compassion, respect, love, and acceptance.

This is one of the biggest discoveries I have made on my journey: I am not my body, whether I am obese or not. Because I defined and judged myself by my body, I went into the world and did the same to others. But we are more than sizes—small, medium, large, and extra-large. Each of us is a being that has no weight or size. How much does a person's humanity weigh? What is the size of our capacity to be channels of compassion, peace, healing, and courage in the world? No scale or BMI can measure this.

You are so much more than your body. You are your words, your ideas, and your actions. You are your heart and spirit, and your deepest thoughts and feelings. No person is human in the unique way that you are. You are filled with courage, humour, purpose, compassion, love, and intelligence. There is no photograph or selfie that can capture the worlds of beauty, goodness, love, creativity, brilliance, magic, and mystery within each of us. Whatever our body appearance, we are all human and members of one human family.

Every day we see filtered and photoshopped images of perfect bodies we can never have. We are convinced that our bodies are who we are. Passing through puberty into adulthood, through middle age and our senior years, we waste so much time lamenting the size of our hips, sagging parts, the grey in our hair, and the lines on our face. The secret to life is not weight loss pills and cosmetic surgery. We never seem to learn the simple truth that there never was or is or will be a perfect body.

Naomi Wolf wrote in her book *The Beauty Myth*, "She wins who calls herself beautiful and challenges the world to change to truly see her." In the 20th century we have been obsessed with thin bodies. In the past 50 years, taste in physical beauty has shown a marked rejection of the curvaceous body—or, to put it bluntly, fat. The appearance of the human body has obviously changed very little through history, but the image of the ideal body has changed a great deal. There was a period when men and women of substantial weight represented abundance, happiness, good health, and desirability. Thinness of body signified poverty, disease, and old age. It also meant spiritual poverty and moral insufficiency. A thin body was considered unlovely.

Today, slimness represents youthfulness, something which we view as highly desirable. But, in earlier centuries, youth was represented by plumpness, physical abundance, and satisfaction. Youthful skinniness or boniness was an indication of sickness, and a lack of fortune, muscle, will, and enthusiasm. Today, we spend money, time, and energy trying to look slim and bony. Fatness and softness, once status symbols for centuries, are now rejected in favour of thinness.

Either way, our shape or weight is irrelevant. What matters most is love, and weight has nothing to do with love. Love is our greatest need and desire. We are all worthy of receiving love, and love is the greatest power we have. No matter how we look, or our waist size, we can all be, receive, and express love at any moment. Our deepest work is to remove the barriers we have built inside ourselves against love. Love is our highest calling, and love, whether giving it or receiving it, always transforms.

None of us is too far gone to be transformed by love. Over time, I realized that all the people who had victimized me were people who had been hurt and wounded themselves and needed love. That doesn't excuse what they did, but it helped me to see them through eyes of compassion.

The cornerstone of wholeness is loving ourselves. The person who most needed my love was myself. I had to learn to love myself enough to take the actions required for my health and wellbeing. Enough to cut myself loose from the shame-based lies I adopted about my identity and worth. Enough to heal from the wounds of my past. Enough to let go of my bitterness and resentment. Enough to forgive myself. Enough to move on. Enough to acknowledge and celebrate what makes me a beautiful human being. Enough to set a high standard for my relationships. Enough to free my heart, spirit, mind, and body. Enough to have confidence, respect, and trust in myself. Enough to take responsibility for my happiness and wellbeing.

I had to love myself that much, and this love within me was big enough to do it.

Chapter Twenty-Three
Blue Lake

The poet Wallace Stevens wrote, "Perhaps the truth depends on a walk around the lake." I've been walking the Blue Lake for over 20 years. Each time, I understand a little more about myself and my life.

The Blue Lake is a volcanic crater lake in South Australia that formed some 28,000 years ago. The lake is known for its famous colour change. From November to March, it turns to a vibrant cobalt blue colour, and then returns to a colder steel grey from April to October. The surface of the lake is 95 feet (29 metres) below the level of the main street of the nearby town, Mount Gambier, and supplies its drinking water.

For years I had driven past the lake, never stepping on the path that circled it. Sometimes I would sit in my car eating and watch the walkers pass by. I envied them, but I was too afraid to walk it myself because of my appearance. Even if I had tried, I was in no condition to do it.

But it is now one of my regular daily walks and one of my favourite places to walk. The path around the lake is a 2.25-mile (3.6 kilometre) loop. People walk or jog, some bring their dogs. Friends and families walk together, then there are those like me who usually walk alone. The path has various places to view the lake and is lit at night.

The lake is surrounded with native and introduced trees. Wallabies, a native of this part of Australia, can often be seen hopping through the foliage around the lake, and feeding on the grass near the pumping station which feeds water to the town. Superb blue fairy-wrens and red-browed finches dart and flutter among the branches and in and out of the fence which protects the lake. I enjoy photographing the lake and its surrounds as I walk. I share these on a Facebook page called "I love Mount Gambier".

The Blue Lake has been my sanctuary. Here I can experience solace and serenity. There is a charm to the Lake. Each walk is a new experience of colours, scents, sounds, and textures. Walking the loop is a place of therapy where I search and examine my soul as I walk. It gives me space to let go of my pain and enjoy nature's beauty while I walk myself to health.

Although I often walk alone, I don't feel sad or lonely. Instead I find it refreshing. I enjoy being by and with myself—alone with my thoughts, alone with my heart, and with the presence of peace, joy, and love. There is a simple, uncomplicated beauty and freedom in nature.

Over time the faces I meet on the trail have become familiar. I'm not the only one who finds the Blue Lake a favourite walking spot. As we pass one another I cheerily say "Howdy!" or "G'day!" with a heartfelt smile. Many times, we stop and chat. I am grateful to walk. This simple privilege has evaded me most of my life.

Many have found inspiration in my determination. When I first started walking the Blue Lake, I had lost a considerable amount of weight, but I was still obese. The regular walkers have witnessed the changes to my body, and some stop to encourage me.

On one walk, a middle-aged woman stopped me on the trail and said I was an inspiration to her. She was overweight herself and told me that she was trying to get healthy and lose weight. I shared with her some of my journey. I told her she was doing an amazing job and that doing this alone was a big thing. I encouraged her to not stress over her weight, but to rather focus on her health.

The woman seemed elated by my words and thanked me. She gave me a hug, and said softly, "Thank you, Jenny. Thank you so much."

People have often said how inspiring I am, and my closest friends are proud of me. It is exciting to give something of worth to others and to make a difference in their life by simply being me. This is in stark contrast to my past where I was a burden to others. Mum made it clear that I was a frustration to her and wasn't shy about holding me responsible for her unhappiness.

I like to think that my journey has not been wasted. Pain has taught me many things. Instead of becoming bitter, I have tried to understand the motives of those who once taunted me. But this could only happen through self-awareness. Years of introspection have given me insight into my own motives; this has given me empathy for others, confidence in myself, and forgiveness for myself.

Although I cannot control others, I can control my own responses. It has helped me offer care to others and give the same compassion I have learned to give myself. People were attracted to this, so I used this understanding to make connections with those I met on the path around the lake.

Connection with people was difficult for me at first. I was always waiting for someone to judge me just as I had always been judged. I feared that if someone was showing me interest, they were simply pacifying or tolerating me. As I walked away, I would worry that I was being criticised or mocked. Perhaps I looked stupid, or silly to others.

There were still those who avoided me like the plague, didn't speak a word, and gave me looks of disapproval. Some of them treated me like I was incompetent, patronized me, and obviously viewed me as inferior.

Becoming more assertive, communicating, and expressing myself was not easy. The opinion of an obese person is usually regarded as inferior to others. I guess it seems that we have nothing of value to say because we can't control our eating habits. Or, that we have a mental weakness so our opinion could not have any substance to it. Many times, people would play the fat card when I said something they didn't like or gave a different point of view. Who was I as an obese person to disagree with another person's opinion, particularly a thin person?

But BMI classification or weight has no effect on competency and intelligence. Some of the greatest, most accomplished, and brilliant human beings throughout history were fat. Notable historical figures such as Socrates, Winston Churchill, and Ben Franklin; successful business leaders like Steve Ballmer; authors like Alfred Hitchcock; iconic musicians like Aretha Franklin; current musicians like Kelly Clarkston; and entertainers like Kevin James, Kathy Bates, John Candy, and Rebel Wilson have and did struggle with obesity. Even Buddha is described as overweight, representing contentment.

My life experiences and the prevalent fat-bias in society were losing their grip over my life. I was having too many positive encounters with people at the Blue Lake and other areas of my life to believe I was the incompetent and useless person I once thought I was.

As my confidence increased, so did my hardy sense of humour. Albeit, slightly twisted and dark at times, I could naturally make people laugh. The better I felt about myself, the more I found in life to laugh about. Tough times taught me not to take situations too seriously and I found humour where others didn't. People who know me would say I am witty and funny. Humour makes me feel good. It helps me overcome my depression and buffers my stress. In my interactions with others I noticed that it did the same for them, and it brought about trust between us. There's something about laughing which draws us closer to one another.

"Laughter," theologian Karl Barth said, "is the closest thing to the grace of God." And Holocaust survivor Viktor Frankyl wrote, "I never would have made it if I could not have laughed."

Laughter is strong medicine. It is good for our body both physically and emotionally. Laughter releases stress which lessens the load on our body, improving our immune system, lifting our mood and reducing pain. A good laugh is a quick way to bring our mind and body back into balance. Humour lightens our burdens, gives us hope, connects us to others, and helps us release negative emotions.

Like others who struggle with their weight, I had low self-confidence because I believed there was something intrinsically wrong with me. After all, a 'normal' person wouldn't get this fat! I believed that I didn't have any special qualities, talents, or abilities. But obesity does not prevent us from having any trait or skill that could be found in a thin person.

What truly makes the world go around are people with big hearts; people who are empathic and compassionate; people who offer listening, acceptance and understanding to others; people who relate to others from a place of authenticity and depth; and people who make us laugh. These are the true traits that make a difference, and these are what the world needs.

Some close and meaningful friendships grew with those I met at the lake. This conflicted with my old beliefs. During these times, I reminded myself that these relationships were mutually beneficial, and that these friends reciprocated out of choice and not obligation. My chronic fear of rejection and abandonment did not die easily, and at times I had to catch myself from becoming too dependent and clingy. It was all part of my journey.

Coming out of obesity is not primarily about losing weight. For me it was developing a new kind of relationship with every part of myself—my thoughts and feelings, my beliefs and attitudes, my physical and mental health, and my relationships with others—my entire outlook on myself and life.

As I changed as a person, and became healthier in my relationships, so did the type of people with whom I related. I made some friends and lost some, including some truly close friendships. Initially, I made friends with people who identified with my pain. But as more healing and freedom unfolded in my life, some of these friends felt threatened and the relationship faded. I still grieve friends I've lost. But my relationship with Fee did not falter. We had our ups and downs, but our bond of love has held us together through thick and thin.

Facing the countless ways obesity damaged me and my life was an ordeal. People often ask me, "How did you do it?" I tell them that the only way through for me was to remember that my journey was not about weight loss, but about love. It was about loving myself because it hurt others when I didn't. It was one day at a time, one hour at a time, one small choice at a time, one small step at a time, one small act of courage at a time, one setback at a time, one realization at a time, one new thought at a time, one conversation at a time, and one belief in myself at a time.

Chapter Twenty-Four

My Life With Doctors

We all like to think we are qualified to give advice. Parenting and weight loss are the most popular topics for this. There is no shortage of people in the world who are not shy about telling others how to raise their children, or how to lose weight. This includes parents, siblings, aunts, cousins, friends, co-workers, neighbours, hairdressers, dentists, fitness junkies, and Facebook friends.

The most common advice I have received from one of these "experts" is that the way to lose weight is to, "eat less and move more." I have made countless attempts to follow this advice and failed countless times. I figured I lacked discipline and willpower.

The "eat less and move more" recommendation promotes outdated and unhelpful ideas about weight loss. It presumes that self-control and exercise are the most important factors to reducing fat. However, research shows that losing weight is much more complicated than that. Obesity and weight loss are extremely complex, involving a range of psychological, physiological, and environmental factors.

It was often assumed by others and myself that I wasn't losing weight because I was not trying hard enough or practicing self-control. After all, it was as simple as counting calories and exercising. But eating is not purely a logical behaviour. We are not robots. While it may be tempting to view our body as a machine, it does not regulate weight simply by "calories in vs. calories out" alone.

We eat for many reasons. Traci Mann, a health psychologist, cites research that tested the common assumption that people with higher self-control are better able to resist junk food. She found that individual levels of self-control didn't make any real difference.

Diet and exercise are important factors of good health, but they are not the main drivers of weight loss. Dieting is like holding our breath. At some point, we have to breathe. Willpower alone is not enough to change and sustain our eating habits. Willpower alone is not enough to maintain a lifestyle of drinking kale smoothies and waking up early to run or go to the gym. Willpower is the ignition that gets a car started, not the fuel that keeps it moving.

The "eat less and move more" approach did great harm to my efforts to overcome obesity. I pushed myself harder and harder at the Blue Lake, frustrated that my weight was not moving, or that my weight loss was slowing down. It wasn't until much later that I realized that, although walking contributed in many ways to my overall health, it was not the sole answer to my weight problem.

Although I lost weight by walking regularly and eating better, this created other health issues for me to address. One day Fee and I were walking together at a nearby national park, and I was feeling oddly tired. As we pushed on, I became unbearably fatigued. My joints and muscles hurt, and every step was painful. In frustration, I slammed my walking stick onto the rocks as I climbed over them. Fee looked back and asked what was wrong. "I don't know. I feel so rotten," I said, as tears welled up in my eyes. My energy was low, and my patience limited. I was exhausted. Every inch of my body ached.

I reasoned that I was just tired and having one of those days. But then the next week I found walking was becoming increasingly difficult. It felt like I might have caught a virus or perhaps had the flu. I was foggy, aching, and fatigued. As each day passed my symptoms worsened. Regular daily activities wore me out. I was always exhausted.

No amount of rest made me feel better. My muscles and joints ached relentlessly. My depression was returning. I reduced my walking, and finally had to stop altogether. Feelings of failure took over me.

Fee ordered some tests, which revealed that I was suffering from adrenal dysregulation (adrenal fatigue), caused by long-term physical and emotional stress. This is a condition in which the adrenal glands are unable to keep pace with the demands of perpetual fight-or-flight arousal. The adrenal glands release the stress hormones cortisol and adrenaline to cope with trauma, increasing heart rate and blood pressure in the process. Eventually, high stress levels can cause our adrenal glands to burn out from overproduction of cortisol. As a result, fatigue sets in.

My life and struggle with obesity, beginning in childhood, was one of constant stress and trauma. I had lived in fight-or-flight mode. Whether it was the trauma I experienced as a child, bullying and persecution at school during my youth, discrimination and harassment in the workplace, or the spiritual abuse I suffered in religion, my adrenal glands were overloaded and depleted with constant demands. Even my efforts to eat healthier and exercise regularly, put stress on my body. From the earliest age, I had lived a sedentary lifestyle and consumed high sugar and processed foods. The transition to more healthy ways of living was a shock to my system.

I realised that addressing my weight meant that things could get worse before getting better. This was true in almost every part of my life—physically, mentally, psychologically, and relationally. Coming out of obesity is filled with ups and downs, peaks and valleys. Being patient, compassionate, and gentle with myself was vital.

Based on Fee's recommendation, I made some dietary changes and added supplements for adrenal support. It wasn't a quick fix, but in time my energy improved and stabilized.

If I had known in advance how hard my journey out of morbid obesity would be, I would have given up much earlier. Little did I realize that adrenal fatigue was the least of my worries.

I went back to walking the Blue Lake, doing two laps each day. I was following a good nutrition plan and began taking antidepressants to manage my depression and hormonal changes. My weight loss accelerated. As it went down, I felt better about myself. The skin around my wrists, elbows and neck turned from brown back to a healthy pink. My rate of perspiration improved, and my left leg shrunk to nearer the size of my right.

There were other, less pleasing consequences of losing weight. My dream as I worked to lose weight, was one of a tighter, toned body. I had not pictured the extra, loose skin. The elasticity of my skin depended on my age. I had been obese since childhood and my skin was not about to shrink to any sort of normality. It didn't matter how I lost weight, whether it was quick or slow. The longer it was stretched out and the older I was, the less likely it was to bounce back. Unfortunately for me, it had taken time to overcome my dysfunctional relationship with myself and the unhealthy lifestyle patterns I had developed.

My loose skin was stretched so far that it would not tighten. When I walked, the skin and fat on my legs moved backward and forward with every step and folded down the centre of each leg. I wore clothes that concealed the flaps of loose skin, including tight undergarments. The loose skin over my lower abdomen would protrude through the leg hole. Rashes and infections developed in the skin folds.

Then, a persistent pain started in my lower abdomen. I reasoned that it was likely hormonal. Meanwhile, my periods returned with a vengeance. Obese women often have abnormal menstrual cycles. Sometimes periods can be very painful. And of course, this is how it was for me. My cramps were so unbearable that it's a miracle that I didn't kill someone in the process.

After talking with Fee, she referred me to a female gynaecologist whose office was in the nearest city a 5-hour drive from home. Being an obese woman increased my risks for numerous health problems treated by obstetricians and gynaecologists, including cancer, in particular endometrial cancer.

The gynaecologist ordered blood tests, which showed that I had an overactive thyroid. In a further scan, it was revealed that the cause was a hot nodule on my thyroid. This was the beginning of my medical education, which became quite extensive.

The overactive thyroid accelerated my body's metabolism, causing weight loss. It was not just my walking and healthier diet that enabled me to drop several clothing sizes and lose weight, it was also my overactive thyroid.

From there it was another long drive to an endocrinologist in the city to deal with my thyroid problem. He assured me that I would not put on weight if the nodule was treated. This is when I learned that there are four things you should never believe that a doctor tells you: "this won't hurt a bit", "I'll be right back", "everything is going to be all right", and "this won't cause you to put on weight".

Radioactive iodine treatment killed the nodule and my thyroid began to slow. But to my horror, I put on weight. My legs swelled with fluid, and the new clothes I had bought no longer fitted. My ankles and feet were swollen, making it harder to walk. My face and stomach ballooned. Despite my vigilance in eating healthier, my weight increased. All the work I had done to that point felt to be slipping away. No matter how hard I tried, I could not lose weight, and only seemed to keep putting it on.

On my return visit to my gynaecologist, she was visibly annoyed by my weight gain. In order to resume my weight loss, she suggested gastric banding, a surgical procedure. The band would constrict my stomach so that I would feel full after eating less food than usual. I declined this treatment because I had already lost a significant amount of weight by my own effort.

With respect to my continuing lower abdomen pain, a date was set for surgery to see if I had endometriosis. Endometriosis is a painful disorder in which tissue similar to that which normally lines the inside of a woman's uterus grows outside the uterus. The symptoms are painful menstrual cramps, intestinal pain, bleeding, and stomach and digestion problems. She explained that a laparoscopy was the necessary surgery to look inside my pelvic area to see endometriosis tissue, and the only way of determining if I had it. I could sense her hesitation as she talked about the surgery. Her discomfort at facing the task of operating on someone who was obese was clear.

A week later I received a call from the gynaecologist. Apprehensive and apologetic, she informed me that she would not be able to perform the surgery. I was too obese. The beds at the treating hospital were not big enough, and I was considered a high risk for complications during surgery. Performing surgery on an obese person would put her at risk of litigation. She recommended I visit another gynaecologist who had, "more experience with someone of my size."

I wanted to scream, but I controlled myself. I wanted to say that my family wouldn't care if I died, my friends were not the suing type, and I'd be dead so I couldn't take her to court. But I knew there was no way of changing her mind. I was a risk that she did not want to take.

So now I was off to a fat woman's gynaecologist, in the same city, five hours from home, who happened to be a man. For medical professionals touted as having expertise "with someone my size", they certainly didn't have the bedside manner to match. As the nurse weighed me, I felt her judgement. Walking into the gynaecologist's consulting room, his disdain was palpable. Fear seized me as I forced myself into the chair beside his desk, which wasn't made for "someone my size."

Gravely looking over my results he said the blood test showed slightly raised cholesterol levels and I should work on this. I explained that I had lost a great deal of weight and spoke of my efforts, but he didn't acknowledge my words. I even showed him a picture of myself before weight loss, but he was unmoved.

I timidly asked that I not be told my weight. My focus had shifted from a number on a scale to making better choices about my physical and mental health. He wasn't pleased with my request. He said gruffly, "Well, it's up to you if you want to take it on board." I had been crammed into his box of the stereotypical obese patient who is unmotivated, lazy, irresponsible, eating all the wrong foods, and not exercising.

At the end of the consult, he handed me a script for some more blood tests. When I left his office, I looked down at the script. There it was, in big, bold letters, my weight. I was devastated.

If a medical professional wants to respectfully and effectively work "with someone my size", they should:

Express a supportive and affirming attitude, recognizing that it's likely to be a distressing experience for an obese person to see a doctor.

Approach the obese patient from a place of not knowing, and setting aside all judgment, assumptions, and stereotypes.

Take the time to inquire and listen to an obese person summarize their history of obesity, and their current progress and challenges.

Refrain from relating to the obese patient as a child, dumb, or inferior.

Interact with the obese patient with the respect, dignity, empathy and compassion that every human being deserves.

That appointment was a major psychological setback for me. It pulled me back down into feelings of self-hatred and despair. The next week I saw my regular doctor. He caringly listened to what had happened and was not surprised. I was not the first to have gone through this. He told me the story about another of his obese patients who had gone to an orthopaedic surgeon to have surgery on his leg. The man could not exercise unless the leg was fixed. The surgeon was insensitive and unsympathetic and would not operate because of the health risk. Like me, the patient had fallen into dejection after seeing the surgeon.

After telling this story, my doctor looked at me with tenderness and compassion in his eyes and said, "I'm sorry you had to experience what you did." Then he paused and a more serious and resolute expression filled his face. He said empathically, "You have lost your focus." And, in a believing manner, "You need to get back to your goal."

Instead of giving me a lecture, he showed he believed in me. I had been stepped on many times in my life. I didn't need someone to put me down, but someone to lift me up.

My doctor knew of a local gynaecologist, and to whom he referred his patients. I made an appointment with the new gynaecologist. So, this would now be my third gynaecologist. But this time it was different. He was respectful, warm, casual, and funny. I took an instant liking to him. He was fine with doing the laparoscopic surgery in the local hospital which did not have wider beds for "someone my size". But no endometriosis was found.

My abdominal pain continued and worsened. It hindered my walking. Sometimes it was so bad that I could not concentrate. At times, it brought me to tears.

King Solomon in the Old Testament Book of Ecclesiastes wrote, "There is a time for everything." He goes on …

> "… time to be born and a time to die,
> a time to plant and a time to uproot,
> a time to kill and a time to heal,
> a time to tear down and a time to build,

a time to weep and a time to laugh,
a time to mourn and a time to dance,
a time to scatter stones and a time to gather them,
a time to embrace and a time to refrain from embracing,
a time to search and a time to give up,
a time to keep and a time to throw away,
a time to tear and a time to mend,
a time to be silent and a time to speak,
a time to love and a time to hate,
a time for war and a time for peace."

Oddly enough, these words describe my journey out of obesity. I have one more to add to the list: a time to scream and a time to stop screaming.

Chapter Twenty-Five
What if I Fall?

Beads of sweat rolled down my face and onto my gown. My heart pounded like a freight train and my stomach felt as if a swarm of locusts was buzzing around in it. Fear had gripped me. What if I made a fool of myself? What if I was mocked for how I looked? It wasn't too late to escape with gown and all, and never look back.

As I sat waiting to be called on stage to receive my master's degree my thoughts were: What if I trip as I walk across the stage? What if I have a coughing fit? What if I drop the certificate?

The moment finally came: "Jennifer Marshall, Master's in Business Administration". When I stepped onto the stage, a massive roar erupted from the audience. Eight of my friends attended the graduation. Jane had the loudest voice and spurred on the crowd. Many knew me from walking the lake or around town. They had seen my perseverance as I worked to become more fit and lose weight. It was nice to be celebrated. The Vice Chancellor handed me my degree, which I did not drop, and shook my hand. He said, "Congratulations, Jennifer. You have done well."

Joy filled my heart as I took the piece of paper. I never heard my father say these words. There is still a little girl inside me who wishes she could have made her dad proud. If only he had told me this. I so wanted him to appreciate me, to want me, to respect me.

Developing self-respect was liberating for me. As I grew and healed so did my pride and confidence in myself, increasing with each step in my journey of a thousand miles. Every action I took, every time I faced my fears, every time I bounced back, and every step outside my comfort zone, was another step on the path of self-respect. I learned that self-acceptance and self-love were expressions of self-respect because I believed I was worth giving these to myself.

Coming out of obesity is not an easy task. My self-acceptance had to be strong enough to overcome the cultural pressure which had kept me obese. Like everyone who struggles with obesity, I was taught to shame myself into weight loss. However, this shame eroded my self-confidence and self-acceptance, and diminished my ability to remain on the weight loss path.

Despite all the ups and downs, my persistence paid off. As my self-confidence improved, so did my job opportunities. I had been working as a contract accountant for some years. To be a good accountant one must be ethical, organized, meticulous, and a good communicator. As my confidence increased, so did the development of these skills. The skill of accounting came naturally to me. Accounting software, management accounting, and financial forecasting, are a few of the areas I thrived in. I taught my clients how to use software in order to make more strategic and effective use of financial data. I created spreadsheets and databases to assist their work productivity.

One of the common myths about accountants is that we are boring people. However, rock star Mick Jagger studied accounting and finance on a scholarship at the London School of Economics. John Grisham has an accounting degree. Mixed Martial Arts icon, Chuck Liddell, is a trained accountant. John Pierpont (J.P.) Morgan's career began as an accountant in 1857.

Itzahk Stern, accountant and friend to Oskar Schindler, is credited with typing the list known as "Schindler's list", which contained the names of Jews who survived the Holocaust because of their employment under Schindler. Itzhak forged documents to classify otherwise "nonessential" Jewish workers as experienced machinists and factory operators in order to protect them from execution. Around 1,100 Jews were saved in this way by the end of the war.

The manager of one of my contract jobs asked if I was interested in tutoring and lecturing at the local university. He said I would be excellent at teaching subjects in IT, maths, finance, and accounting.

I was caught off-guard by this invitation. It confronted the old story which had burdened me all my life. My lifelong shame filter through which I saw myself had blinded me to my gifts and skills. People often saw potential in me that I could not see for myself as they were buried beneath layers of self-doubt.

The Jenny-is-no-good story was familiar. It was a self-condemning identity which had been programmed into me from childhood and governed my life. I didn't question it or have to think about it, I just fell in line with the script I knew. Whenever it was challenged by someone who saw good in me, I felt threatened.

Marianne Williamson wrote, "Our deepest fear is not that we are inadequate. Our deepest fear is that we are powerful beyond measure. It is our light, not our darkness that most frightens us. We ask ourselves, 'Who am I to be brilliant, gorgeous, talented, fabulous?' Actually, who are you not to be?"

We tend to believe that what we fear is not being enough, not being adequate, and failing. Most of us accept that this is what stops us in life. However, Williamson states that while we might believe this is true, the real reason we fail to reach our dreams is because we fear our brilliance.

I painfully realized that I had been locked away from my true self by those who had shamed me. But when I stepped back, I realised that my jailer changed faces; it was now me. My Jenny-is-bad story kept the belief that I was inadequate going. It protected me from stepping outside my comfort zone and risking failure. This story kept me from taking responsibility for my potential.

I understand the "Who am I …?" question. Often, I would say to myself: Who am I to be someone of worth, to lose weight, to believe I have potential, be happy, make a difference, write a book, teach at a university? As my self-acceptance increased, I questioned the old story. My internal dialogue changed to, "Maybe I could be?" and "If others can, why can't I?"

As my first day of teaching approached, I stressed; sleep eluded me the night before. Although my lecture and tutorial were prepared, I was nervous. For a woman who had been in the spotlight as the target of ridicule, the thought of being the focus of attention in front of a class of students was frightening.

I perspired profusely, my muscles were tight with tension, and moving about the classroom was awkward. But as I confronted my fears they dissipated, my confidence climbed, and I enjoyed it.

Being myself worked perfectly with my students. My life hardships translated into being a more real person with them. My quirky sense of humour was accepted and encouraged. The trauma I had experienced in my life gave me natural empathy and understanding for my students. I connected with their struggles inside and outside the classroom. I knew what it was like to feel dumb, slow and down on myself, and constantly reminded that I was incapable. This fuelled me to encourage and inspire my students. I came to love them. We had a bond. Teaching drew me out of myself and my self-consciousness decreased in the classroom.

My classes included adult learners in their 40s and 50s who were studying to start a new career or make a better life for themselves. Most of them were working against major obstacles in their life. I understood. It had been a hard road pushing uphill to improve my own life.

I consider myself a late bloomer … a really late bloomer. In many ways I feel like I am just getting started in my life and my best days are still ahead of me. It is exciting. I was dealt a crappy hand of cards, but I have chosen to use those cards in a positive way. We all have the same starting point, where we are right now, and we have the rest of our lives left.

Nurturing my students came naturally for me. I wanted them to know that they could do well if they believed in themselves. In class I would share stories from my own life, and how unlikely it was that I would ever succeed in academics. I told my students I believed in them. In time I was asked to teach more courses in maths, business, and finance.

Maths doesn't come easy for many. I encouraged patience and persistence. One student, Shelly, could not grasp how to calculate fractions. Reluctantly, she asked me for help. Shelly explained that she was hopeless at maths but wanted to pass. It had taken a few tutorials to develop trust between us. I thought the concepts were too abstract for her and if I showed her how fractions related to her everyday life, she would catch on.

We sat together and drew pictures of pies to illustrate halves and quarters and eighths. I showed her what a half of a half a pie looked like through a drawing, then I explained the maths behind it. She understood it. Shelly was so excited. I saw her confidence grow from that moment. Soon, she was helping another student understand fractions, and then she explained it to the rest of the class.

Christopher Robin's words of wisdom to Winnie-the-Pooh apply to all of us, "You are braver than you believe, stronger than you seem, and smarter than you think." Sometimes we just need an understanding and nurturing ally to draw us out.

When we are wounded, we need someone to believe in us before we can believe in ourselves. This was true in my journey. Even my teaching position was the result of someone else's belief in me, as I could not believe in myself. One of the greatest gifts we can give another is to see their brilliance and reflect it back to them.

A university senior academic, Jane, encouraged me to teach a master's level class and join a graduate program for managers. I loved Jane. She was an intelligent, affirming, and caring woman. Jane was my rock as I stepped back into the world of academics. She encouraged me to pursue my MBA.

Although I had taught undergraduates, teaching master's level classes seemed a huge step. These would be students who had qualifications and experience in their field. But Jane had confidence in me, so, I did.

As I worked toward my MBA, I discovered it was not as difficult as I had expected. It was a lot of work, but I thrived in my studies and projects. Throughout my years of education, I believed I was unintelligent and incompetent. Completing the master's degree drew out my ability to think critically and deeply, as well as articulate and write. My work experience gave me confidence to analyse subjects and theories and show how they related to the real world of business and finance.

This Jenny was a completely different person than the one who was beaten down by her childhood, youth, and early adulthood experiences. This meant that whenever I returned to my childhood home to visit my father and sisters, I felt like an alien. My family related to me the same way they always had, with indifference and insult. They could not accept the new person I had become, and I was no longer the person they needed me to be.

I had to give up my life as I knew it to find a new one, to relinquish everything I was clinging to and begin again. I couldn't go back to the way it was because I had outgrown it and it no longer worked. In order to fly, I had to give up what weighed me down. Time doesn't necessarily heal our pain. We must learn to live our best life in spite of it.

On the day of my graduation when my name was called, it was both unnerving and liberating. In the audience there were friends who had become my family. They came to share and celebrate this milestone with me. Several of my undergraduate students were also present to receive their undergraduate degree. Of course, there was Jane with a beaming smile shining from her face and a big voice cheering me from the crowd.

We all fall sometimes. I fell many times in my journey. But falling isn't always a bad thing. Sometimes when you fall, you fly.

Chapter Twenty-Six
Under the Scalpel

Barry had been a part of my life for over 40 years. We grew up together. He was there when I was mocked at school and ostracised by my peers. Over time our bond had become so deep that I could not tell where he ended, and I began. We were inseparable, both emotionally and physically. He gave me comfort and security. I used him as an excuse for my failures and assumed he was the reason for my rejection.

The decision to separate from him was difficult and I felt his loss deeply. Removing him from my life was traumatic. I grieved his loss and our relationship. It took some time to learn how to live without him, and to this day there are times that I still miss him, and I imagine he is with me.

Barry was a flap of loose, sagging skin, hanging from my abdomen. By shedding a massive amount of weight, I was left with a large mass of excess skin and fat. It was unsightly, embarrassing, and interfered with many of my daily activities. It required careful cleaning beneath the folds of skin to prevent infection and painful rashes. Despite my health improvements, I never felt comfortable in my body. As my best efforts to lose weight could not remove this excess, I began to lose motivation.

One Saturday evening Fee gave me a leaflet, which had come across her desk at the clinic. It advertised a group of plastic surgeons in a nearby town who did procedures such as abdominoplasty. This surgery removes the excess skin from the abdominal region after substantial weight loss. It includes liposuction to remove fat cells from the area.

I looked at her, confused. Why was she showing me this? Surely, I was still too fat to consider it.

Bewildered, I said, "I thought you told me I shouldn't have this done?"

Fee said, "No, I've never said that."

The truth is that I had been too fearful to consider the surgery, and too ashamed to face it.

I said, "I thought I was too fat!"

"Not necessarily," said Fee.

"Huh? Are you telling me to get it done?", my heart was beating fast.

She said, "I'm just showing you the medical interventions they are offering elsewhere. These are the types of procedures you might want to consider."

I asked, "Should I get it done?"

"That's up to you," she said.

I was totally unprepared for this. The conversation moved on, but I kept thinking about it. Despite my fear, I knew it was necessary. The excess skin would never go away on its own. It could only be removed through surgery.

The next week I made an appointment with Dr. Todd and told him about the idea. Without hesitation he asked, "Would you like me to write the referral letter?" Stunned, I was confronted by the response.

Dr. Todd said he had thought it would be a good idea, but he didn't want to push it. He believed that when I was ready for this step, I would tell him. I should have kept my mouth closed! Fear clutched at my heart like a vice, but I knew I should take this step.

The persistent, steady sense of love which had pervaded my heart for so long was now nudging me forward in another direction.

So, I said yes. It was a terrified yes, but a yes, nonetheless.

Fee researched and gave me a list of surgeons she thought would be right for me. I chose a female. If I was going to get this done, I didn't want some unknown man seeing this most shameful part of my naked body. Dr. Todd wrote my referral letter without hesitation. The next morning, I made an appointment for a consultation with the surgeon, which was scheduled for a Saturday. It was a long drive from my hometown to the city.

When I arrived at the clinic, I nervously spoke with a receptionist who gave me some forms to complete. I then took a seat in the waiting area. Soothing music was playing, and soft abstract art hung on the walls.

Waiting to be called, I had plenty of time to ponder the endless possibilities. What would this surgeon say to me? What if she shamed or belittled me? What if she rejected me? What if I was put through the same trauma I experienced with that gynaecologist? By the time I had worked myself into a frenzy of fear, my name was called.

The surgeon greeted me, "Hi, Jenny. I'm Dr. Anderson." She was a serious but softly spoken lady. In the first part of our consultation she asked me a range of questions about my health, medical history, and weight loss. I showed her a picture on my phone, which had been taken when I was close to 600 pounds. She listened intently and empathically as I shared my journey. I explained how long I had been working to lose weight through regular exercise and healthy eating.

She said, "It can be hard to lose weight. Sometimes we find that removing excess flesh can help with weight loss." I had never heard this before. It was music to my ears!

Dr. Anderson asked me to stand so she could look at the fold of skin on my lower abdomen. Surprisingly, it was just a matter of fact for her. She gently lifted the loose skin and took a quick look. She then weighed me, without judgement.

We sat down again, and she ran through the procedure, including the risks. She explained that this was major surgery. I was morbidly obese, there could be complications, including the possibility of scarring, hematoma, infection, seroma, blood clots, wound healing problems, and risks related to anaesthetic. I would need to have calf compressors on my legs during the operation and afterwards to prevent thrombosis.

The rewards of the surgery and removal of my excess skin would improve my quality of life significantly. Sitting back, she said, "Something for you to think about. Contact me if you want to proceed."

I left the building, and sat in the car, thinking about our conversation. My emotions were conflicted. I was afraid, yet I knew this surgery would make a real difference to my life. It offered hope in my relentless efforts to lose weight. I wanted this flap of skin and fat taken from my body. But it was clear that there were serious risks related to this surgery, especially for someone like me. Yet, Dr. Anderson was willing to go ahead with it. She had not hesitated.

I texted Fee and a few other close friends to tell them that the appointment went well. My phone rang almost instantly. It was Fee, "Do it! If you feel okay about it, it's time to do it." This was the same sentiment of all my friends. Although it was my decision, I needed their morale support to get through this. Knowing they were behind me was the last little push I needed. Still sitting in the car in the clinic car park, I dialled their number to inform them of my decision. The answer was, yes. The surgery was scheduled for two months' time.

Fee and I had decided beforehand to take a holiday together to Victoria to rest and relax. It was a 6-hour drive from the city in South Australia to regional Victoria where we were holidaying.

By the time I arrived my stomach was in knots and I felt violently ill. The strain of the decision had taken a toll. I was beset by worry. What if my weight was a problem for the anaesthetist and they would not operate on me? Obese patients have a much higher risk of airway problems during a general anaesthetic. What if the surgery didn't go well and one of the many risks occurred? Fee calmed me down. She said that if Dr. Anderson was willing to go ahead, then she was confident that the surgery would be successful. To further calm my nerves, I called the clinic and expressed my concerns about the anaesthetic. I was given a number and spoke directly with the anaesthetist's clinic. A nurse assured me that my weight would not be a problem.

All the lights were green. I called the surgery a "Barry-ectomy". I got a lot of mileage out of this. I told people that the decision to remove Barry was "gut-wrenching" and I had grown sick and tired of him "hanging around all the time", and how it was time to "completely cut" Barry and our co-dependent relationship out of my life, and "I would be gutted".

My friends continued their support as the day of the surgery drew closer. There were anxious moments but getting everything in place beforehand was a useful distraction. My friend, Joy, recorded Barry White songs in honour of my upcoming Barry-ectomy. As we travelled together back to the city for the impending surgery, we sang to the songs she had recorded.

I barely slept the night before. It was my first major surgery. Fasting wasn't a problem as I didn't want to eat anyway. Joy drove me to the hospital. Checking-in at the front desk, I noticed that everyone around was slim in comparison to me. I tried not to think about the surgery or what would be seen of my naked body.

At the reception, my details were taken, and we were led to a waiting room. After a while we were taken to another room where I was asked to undress and put on a gown. I was weighed, again. The nurse rubbed an iodine solution on my skin in the area of the surgery. This involved lifting Barry to swab beneath the thick layer of skin and fat. It was painful for me to face this. I had done my best to hide Barry from the world, now he was fully exposed to someone I did not know.

When Dr. Anderson arrived, she marked my body with a green marker, so she knew where to make the cuts during the surgery. She lifted Barry again. The area was moist from the iodine. I blamed myself as the marker did not work. Sensing my discomfort, she spoke gently to me, explaining what she was doing and why. She asked me to stand so she could photograph the area she was about to remove. I awkwardly stood there.

At that point, Joy was still with me. We joked about Barry to relieve my tension. I did my best to maintain a sense of humour, but there was no suppressing the gravity of the situation. So many painful memories had been etched into this mass of excess skin. Removing Barry was another death necessary for me to gain my life.

The anaesthetist walked in as we were laughing. I explained my Barry-ectomy humour, and she laughed with us. She went through all the details about the anaesthetic process.

Then I waited and waited and waited. We had arrived at 12 pm, and Joy stayed with me until about 5 pm. I made several trips to the bathroom to relieve my anxious bladder. As I waited, my fears increased. I was not concerned about dying, but about the shame I felt. The thought of being alone with medical staff peering at this part of my anatomy terrified me. But there was no turning back now. At 6.30 pm they finally called me into surgery. It had been a long wait, not just the previous 6 and a half hours, but to get to this point in my life.

I was wheeled to the waiting area outside the operating theatre, the nurse introduced herself and made me comfortable. She told me Dr. Anderson would be getting me soon, and she left. As I waited, I could hear the anaesthetist and Dr. Anderson talking. The nurse returned and wheeled me into the operating theatre. Dr. Anderson greeted me with a big beautiful smile on her face, "Here she is!"

As I lay on the table, the anaesthetist introduced me to the nurses. At the same time a nurse attached calf compressors to my legs. Dr. Anderson walked me through the details of the surgery, indicating that she did not anticipate any problems. She asked me if I had any questions, which I didn't.

The anaesthetist placed the mask over my face and asked me to count backwards. I fell asleep.

My memory of that moment is one of peace and love. The warm, blissful and radiant love emanated from within me and saturated every molecule of my being. It felt familiar, close, and freeing. In those moments it was as if the barrier between the physical and spiritual worlds became whisper-thin and connected through love.

It was so beautiful.

Chapter Twenty-Seven

Life After Barry

"Wakey, wakey. It's all over now," a male voice said cheerfully, rousing me from my haze.

My groggy eyes had barely opened, and the voice spoke again, "Hello, Jennifer. You are in recovery. Can you tell me what procedure you had done?" Even in my daze, my sense of humour was not far from me. "I've had a Barry-ectomy" I answered with a half-smile on my face. "We've got a live one here! Wheel her down to ICU," he said.

Rolling down the hallway, still half asleep, I tried to grasp what just happened. I had no idea how much this surgery would change my life. As my bed was pushed into the ICU, I noticed that the sides were up. In my delirium, I imagined being in a crib as a child. This was not a soothing thought. I was sexually abused as a toddler. Being violated as a vulnerable child by those I trusted left a deep wound in my soul. There is no room for recovery from this.

My lower abdomen, where Barry had been, was uncomfortably tight. I was too afraid to touch it. For most of my life I hated my body. Now, I was frightened of it. I could not bring myself to look at the demolition done to my abdomen. When nurses came to tend my scars and stitches, I turned away so I could not see it.

My first night in recovery I had my own nurse, Kim. Physically, we could have not been more different. I was Australian, she was Asian. I was big-boned and stocky, she was petite. But I quickly discovered we were both big-hearted. Despite her size, Kim had a big heart which was full of empathy.

Once I regained some coherency, I chatted with Kim. I shared the story which led to the Barry-ectomy. She listened with interest and compassion. I felt seen and heard, without judgment. Kim expressed amazement and admiration. She had genuine respect for me and my story.

Kim anticipated everything I needed. She went to great lengths to make me comfortable and tend to my care. I found this awkward at first being the recipient of genuine care.

There were so many times throughout my childhood and teen years that I needed mum to see me, hear me, care for me, and be my strength. I had always thought it was me. There was something wrong with me, the way I looked, the way I talked, my personality, something was wrong with me. As I grew up, I wanted to help mum because I blamed myself. I thought if I could fix her misery, she'd want me.

The absence of a stable, nurturing relationship with my mother meant I felt cheated. I wanted it to be different. Even after her death, I could not grieve her loss freely because I concluded that I was unworthy of love. I went through cycles of denial, anger, and depression. Once I became healthier inside, I realized that mum's emotional absence was not because something was wrong with me, but something that was broken in her. This freed me to grieve what I never had and make peace with it.

When Dr. Anderson walked into my room the following morning, I asked if she had said goodbye to Barry on my behalf. She laughed and said, "Yes, we said goodbye to him". She explained that she had removed a large amount of flesh, and that I had lost a lot of blood. With a concerned look on her face, she said that it had been a big surgery.

But it would not be my last.

The change to my body was massive. Although I was unable to see the surgery, I could feel that the stitches stretched across my abdomen from the far side of my left hip across to the far side of my right one. The never-ending scar covered more than half of my body. Dr. Anderson had cut out and repositioned my belly button higher up on my abdomen. It took me a while to adjust to its new position. I had been accustomed to it hanging low in the sagging flesh which had been Barry.

For the first time I could remember, I could see my upper thighs, which for most of my life had been hidden beneath excess skin and fat. Without Barry it felt like there was a crater beneath my waist. I had no idea of the extent of the excess skin I had in that area of my body. Dr. Anderson had lifted and tightened the areas where it had been removed. My body felt like it was being delicately held together by rubber bands. A brace for compression was necessary to hold my skin to the muscles beneath.

My new life without Barry made me feel vulnerable. For the first time since childhood, my female anatomy was not buried beneath a flap of fat and skin. It took time for my brain to catch up with the physical change. My mind played tricks on me. I felt itchy as if Barry was still there. Reaching down to scratch beneath the skin folds I discovered they were no longer there. I was stressed about moving too much, fearing I would tear my stitches and come undone.

Although I was slowly coming to terms with the surgery to remove Barry, and joked about the ordeal, it was still a difficult emotional adjustment to no longer have my obesity to hide behind. The Barry-ectomy changed virtually everything in my life.

Being single, I was told that on release from the hospital I should stay with a family member or friend near the surgeon's clinic for a few weeks until I had gained more strength. Fee drove the five hours to the city to see me and pick me up from the hospital. She checked my wound, the surgeon's work, made sure I had all the necessary drugs and supported me as I left the building. She took me to the home of my lifelong friend, Jean, who had insisted that I stay with her. I struggled being on the receiving end of Jean's attention and care. More than once, Jean had to assure me that I was not a burden, and that she was happy to look after me.

There was also a 4-legged assistant that aided my recovery process. Jean set a pillow over my abdomen, so her dog Lucy could lay on my lap without pressing on the area of the surgery. I called her the "Love Machine." Cuddling little Lucy was a genuinely healing experience. She sat on my new lap, taking the place of Barry, and soaked up all the attention I could give her.

I had a couple of follow-up visits to the clinic to examine my wounds, check on my recovery, and eventually remove the stitches. Technically, this was "progress," but my sore, swollen, and bloated body told me otherwise. And I missed Barry.

The clinic nurse understood the magnitude of what I had done. On the second visit she said, "Oh lovey, it's going to be at least twelve weeks before you start feeling human again. You are going to be swollen for a long time. You have had major surgery." Looking back, I can see how I had been in denial. A part of me did not want to accept the extent of what had taken place. This was not going to be a short and sweet recovery, but a long and arduous one.

With extended leave from work, my life revolved around healing my body. There were many dark days in the process of recovery. I was easily fatigued, and the most mundane tasks exhausted me. Getting dressed or showering was like running a marathon. But, despite being cautioned otherwise, I pushed myself. One day I could not stop vomiting from overexertion. I would awaken each day with the optimism of all the things I might try doing and was completely out of energy by the time I had showered and combed my hair.

Showering itself was an ordeal. The wound was protected with surgical dressing, which was to be kept dry, so I could not stand beneath the shower. Jean helped me wash my hair over the trough in her laundry. This brought back memories of mum washing my hair as a child. To wash my body, I stood in the shower over a bucket of water using a face washer to wipe myself clean. But, even with all this effort, I managed to wet the dressing.

After two weeks under Jean's care, I travelled home. The hospital where I had the surgery, my follow-up visits, and my friend Jean, were a five-hour drive. On most occasions, I flew back and forth. It was the little things that felt like major victories, like no longer needing an extension for the seatbelt on the plane.

My close friend, Scott the mechanic, picked me up at the airport on my flight back after the surgery. His response was an indication of how significant the surgery had been. My change in appearance was going to shock a lot of people. He shared his deep admiration for the steps I had taken to address my weight. He told me that he admired me for facing my shame. I didn't feel brave, but he used this to describe me.

A follow-up appointment with Dr. Anderson revealed that I had developed a seroma. Numerous times it was necessary for me to have fluid painfully drained out by needle. Concerned about the possibility of an infection, I was given three rounds of antibiotics.

My weight went down over the months after the surgery. Just as predicted, removing the fat cells caused further weight loss as there was less fat tissue to generate inflammation in my body. The fat tissue in my body had developed in childhood. Obesity in childhood set me up for an unhealthy metabolism throughout my life. Morbid obesity in childhood virtually guaranteed obesity in my adulthood, which was the case for me.

I continued to shed weight in my recovery process but could not buy new clothes until the area had completely healed. In the meantime, my attire was oversized clothes that no longer fitted, and an assortment of bandages, pads, and the surgical brace. The only thing lacking was duct tape.

Slowly, I learned to live without Barry. I had not known life without this excess fat and skin. There were moments when I wished I had never gone through with it. I was stripped of the only identity I ever had. One night in bed at Jean's home, I began to sob. I had spent my entire life hiding behind my obesity, and the story that I was worthless and unlovable. I had mastered that script and role perfectly, but I wasn't sure I could take on the role of confident and capable Jenny.

But as weeks and months progressed, I no longer thought of my surgery as losing something but gaining something. Coming out of obesity was an internal transformation, not an outward and physical one. The most dramatic change was not something determined on a scale but came in the form of a different relationship with me. As difficult as it had been to surgically remove a lifetime of fat and skin, and lose weight, overcoming shame was far more demanding.

A crucial step in my journey of freedom was letting go of Barry. We had spent a lifetime together, surviving and coping one trauma after another. Letting Barry go became a symbol of the psychological and emotional changes that had taken place inside me. Closing the chapter on Barry meant it was time for me to embrace a new life, free from shame.

My appearance had changed dramatically, and it was noticeable to everyone who knew me. When I first drove to the nearby café at the lake for coffee, people I knew looked at me stunned. I understood their silence.

My frightening scar felt more like a badge of honour. I asked one friend if she would like to see it. She gasped at the sight of the scar over half of my body. With a shocked look on her face she said, "Oh my God, Jenny! You poor thing."

Ten months after surgery, Fee and I went to New South Wales where we walked Mount Kosciusko, the highest peak in Australia. I had been gradually doing more walking around the Blue Lake and other trails at home to build up my strength. We took a ski lift to get near to the plateau, from there it was a 7 kilometre walk to the summit, and the same distance back to the lifts—a total of 14 kilometres. Fee had never done this walk herself, and we shared this experience with immense joy and gratitude. We celebrated how far I had come in my healing process.

Coming out of shame and obesity has involved climbing many mountains. Often, the mountains seemed too high and daunting to be conquered. People called me brave and an inspiration. But the way I see it, I just never gave up. Call it determination, persistence or stubbornness, I just kept going. There was life after Barry. He was gone. I was free.

The great ancient Greek historian, Thucydides, wrote, "The secret to happiness is freedom. And the secret to freedom is courage."

Healing, transformation, and overcoming requires courage. There's no way around that. We all have courage, even if we must dig to find it.

Chapter Twenty-Eight
I Am Not a Body

My weight was a symptom of the shame I felt. We can become addicted to alcohol, drugs, fitness, sex, co-dependent relationships, and social media to escape negative feelings such as worthlessness, inadequacy, and rejection. My addiction was food. Rather than lessen my shame, the more I ate the greater it became. This toxic feeling poisoned every part of my life. Every relationship, action, thought, and feeling happened in a space of self-hatred.

We can hide almost every other addiction except the addiction to food. My food addiction was on display for the world to see through my weight. Unfortunately, food addiction and obesity are unforgivable sins in Western society. My life had been plagued with fat-shaming. Sadly, this is still widespread in every culture. Shaming an obese person to manipulate them to lose weight does not work. I have been taunted by this treatment most of my life. There is simply no excuse for being fat, it's all my fault.

But I am more than my body. My body is part of who I am, but it is not all of me. It does not define who I am or determine my worth. This was true when I was at my highest, and when I was at my lowest weight. My true self cannot be measured by the BMI index or the numbers on a scale.

My life had always revolved around my body in the form of food addiction, obesity, fat-shaming, and discrimination. Then came the major changes of exercise, healthy eating, weight loss, surgeries, the admiration of others for losing weight, and the improvement of my health and appearance. The focus had been my body.

But it had been a deeper work which had changed my life. Learning to love myself as I hurt was the real root of this external change. Focussing on my body alone did not acknowledge all that had happened within me. This journey of pain had taught me how to love. It had taught me how to feel and to see beyond my own façade and the façades of others. Over the years leading up to the removal of Barry I had changed as a human being. My motives had moved from self-protection to avoid being hurt, to loving myself and others as freely as I could. My focus changed from getting my own way and manipulating others to get it, to personal integrity and doing the best I could in every situation.

This change had not been an easy process, but the satisfaction I now feel in living this way is worth all the suffering I have endured. There is something deeply satisfying about becoming more of the person you love on the inside. This satisfaction goes beyond how you look and stems from the core of your being.

So now, losing Barry and the new healing it brought was the icing on the cake. It did not satisfy me, but I knew it reflected the transformation that had occurred within me.

Six months after the Barry-ectomy, I returned to the surgeon for a check-up. Despite the size of the seroma, the area had mostly healed. As we discussed the outcome of the last surgery, I mentioned another area which was troubling me. On my upper abdomen, a roll of skin circled around both sides of my body to my back and up under my shoulder blades. I affectionately called the front part of this roll "Vera the Veranda" as she kept my feet dry in the shower. The back portion I named "Wendy the Wings", as she was roughly in the place and shape of wings.

As I discussed this with the surgeon I said, "I can see a lot more now that Barry has gone. I'm going grey!"

Laughing she said, "And you'll see even more when Vera goes!"

Two separate surgeries were required to remove the front and back rolls of excess skin, each requiring a stay in the hospital for three days. After the surgeries, I was disappointed about the size of my chest. Surgery could remove the excess skin and fat, but it could not reduce the size of my chest cavity. I had no idea that my chest was this size under the rolls. Dr. Anderson explained that certain aspects of my body's development were affected by childhood obesity.

Fee's mother came for a visit at the hospital and gave me a shirt from the store I frequented for my clothes. She purchased a size 18. It was my first "slim" shirt. To my surprise it fit!

Jean picked me up at the hospital to take me back to her home to recuperate. On the way, we stopped at a small town in the hills near her home. I was desperate for a real cup of coffee. We drank our coffee under the veranda, outside. Cars sped past, trees rustled in the wind, and birds chirped as they flitted from limb to limb. I soaked it all in as I felt the fresh breeze on my skin.

But something was different. I wasn't sure what it was. There was an unusual stillness in the atmosphere. I felt peaceful. I had always been sensitive to the thoughts and feelings of others, but it was more than that. As I looked around, I noticed others surrounding us under the same veranda enjoying their coffee and eating. Everyone was focussed on their own conversation, chatting over their food.

"No one's staring at me?", I asked Jean.

She looked around, "No, they are not."

"What did they used to say?", I asked.

She considered for a minute, then hesitantly said, "They'd mock and laugh."

This wasn't a revelation to me. I had always been aware of the stares, condemning glances, and mutters of mockery as I walked past. I looked at Jean in sadness and said, "I thought so."

For the first time I could remember, I was physically invisible. I did not stand out, nor was I of interest for my appearance. This meant I could be in public and meld in with the crowd, something I had yearned for. I was no longer a sideshow freak. No one was looking out the corner of their eye to take a quick peek at the fat woman. No one was judging me as lazy, irresponsible, and shameful. The feeling of constant exposure was gone. I was at peace.

It would be a 12-week recovery process after the final surgery before I knew how it all looked. Close to 25 pounds was cut from my body from all three surgeries (Barry, Vera, and Wendy), which represented less than ten percent of the amount of weight I'd lost on my own. But it had made a huge change to my body shape. It was easier to find clothes that fit and looked good on me. My body was in proportion. I no longer needed undergarments to cover the folds of excess skin and fat.

Even with all the weight I lost on my own, and the internal work I had done, the rolls of excess skin had been a constant reminder of my past. Each time I saw my reflection in the mirror I was reminded of the shame where it had all started. This is why these three surgeries were so important for me. It wasn't so others would see me differently, it was so I would see myself differently. It helped me to stop identifying myself with what happened to me in my past. I began to feel that my body reflected who I was on the inside, and I could focus on who I wanted to become.

After these surgeries my arms fell more easily to my sides. When I leaned against the back of a chair, I noticed that the roll on my back was gone. For the first time in my life I discovered I had a waist!

Stepping out beyond the weight of my old appearance was liberating. It was both thrilling and disappointing—thrilling because people treated me with a level of respect and dignity I had not experienced before, and disappointing because one should not have to lose weight to experience this.

Despite the transformation of my body, I'm never going to be a model. I wish I could convince everyone trying to lose weight that the goal is not becoming thin. The goal is to be healthy—physically, mentally, emotionally, and relationally. The goal is to be transformed on the inside so that taking care of our health in all ways is easier.

It had been the perfect storm that formed what my body became. My family had a history of obesity. Mum had gestational diabetes while pregnant with me, which affected my metabolism from a young age, causing me to grow more quickly than others my age. I was genetically dealt a big-boned and broad-shouldered body, thanks to my father. Even my hands and feet were large. Constant family trauma created heightened stress levels which sabotaged my metabolism, encouraging weight gain.

A slender and petite bone structure and body was not the product of my efforts. Sometimes we need to be reminded that there is no ideal woman. Women come in all different shapes, sizes, and colours. What it means to look like a woman is an infinite number of combinations and possibilities. Beauty and femininity cannot be defined by body shape and size. Being attractive as a woman isn't necessarily looking like a model. Full-bodied or plus-size women can be beautiful, sensual, and voluptuous.

Over time, I accepted that these were aspects of my body that I could not change. My stocky and big boned body structure did not make me less feminine. My femininity was as valid and authentic as any other woman. As a woman, appearance alone did not determine my femininity, and being thin was not the only way to be attractive. There are many things which made me a woman, including my desire to love and nurture others. But I could only discover this through love.

Maintaining balance was a struggle at first as my centre of balance had shifted. Losing more weight from the front of my body was disorientating. When I stood up from bending over, I would often feel as if I could fall backwards. It took a while to adjust to the change in weight distribution.

With all the changes happening in my mind and body, my posture improved. Slowly, I began to straighten up. I would never stand perfectly erect, but I was no longer the Hunchback of Notre Dame. It was a difficult process to change my posture, and it hurt physically. My shoulders ached as I worked at it. My lower back felt tight and the muscles at the front of my hips were sore.

I focussed on improving my posture while walking. Instead of walking with my head down, I looked up. Trees were swaying in the wind. Birds were in the trees and wildflowers were blooming amongst the grass on the sides of the trail. At times I could see kangaroos feeding in the distance. It was a different world without shame. Standing and walking in an upright position continued the process of inner healing. I now made more eye contact with others, allowing myself to be seen, and relating to the world from my heart.

But despite all this progress, I was plagued with constant stomach issues. Fee arranged for me to have a food sensitivity test. I received the results one afternoon through an email while at work. Of the 269 foods tested, I was sensitive to 68. And pretty much all of the 68 were staples of my current diet such as milk and milk products, nuts and eggs, potatoes and legumes, olive oil and spices, several fruits that I ate regularly, and a long list of other food items.

This was not a good day for me. I threw a temper tantrum. I cried and I sulked. It just wasn't fair!

Eventually, I forwarded the results to Fee and we spoke about it. She empathised with my disappointment. The next morning when I lifted the blind to look out into the backyard, I noticed some bags on the door mat. Fee had left a stack full of alternative foods. She had bought rice milk, coconut milk, coconut yogurt, gluten-free foods, and several other items from the list of foods I could eat. Her kindness touched me, love filled my heart and hope emerged. In the days and weeks to come I found enjoyment in experimenting with these alternative foods to create tasty meals.

Fee enjoyed my interpretation of old favourites made with the alternative foods and spices I was able to use. I began experimenting with baking breads, biscuits and scones from my list of approved ingredients. I shared my Honey Spice Biscuits at the Blue Lake with some of the regular walkers I knew. I tempered their gratitude by explaining that they were the guinea pigs of a new recipe I had tried. My use of spice to compensate for less sugar was a hit and they proved popular.

Just like Forrest Gump who kept on running, I kept cooking. There was Jenny's Vegetable Scones, Jenny's Tandoori Pizza, Jenny's Salmon Salad, Jenny's Beef and Vegetable Pasta sauce, and on it went. I share these recipes with people all over the world through my website and social media.

It took time for my body to adjust to the new diet. Little by little I noticed several improvements to how I felt physically. The first was an increased release of fluid. The pain in my stomach stopped, my joints felt better, and my recurring headaches went away. I lost more weight. Walking was easier, my concentration improved, and my moods stabilized. Living inside my obese body had been physically painful and hampered my everyday life. It was liberating to feel well inside my body. I looked healthy and my skin radiated. My outlook on life changed, life was good. People who knew me commented on my health which could be seen in my appearance.

Over forty years of public shame and humiliation had come to an end. I had no idea that it would change this quickly because of the cut from a surgeon's scalpel. It felt too easy after all those years of hard work. It was almost disillusioning. My constant efforts to prove my worth had failed to change how others saw me, but surgery had the power to do so.

The transformation of my body confirmed that pinning my identity and value on my weight was futile. Many thin people hate themselves and feel worthless, while many overweight people are happy and free inside themselves. We are wrong to assume that all models are brimming with self-confidence, inner peace, and self-love.

In the end, it doesn't matter what anyone else says about who we are, but what we know about ourselves. For me this involved unlearning many false things I had been told by others, beginning as a child. The question of who I am could not be answered through my body. Instead, I discovered my true self through love.

I understand that you are in pain, but that pain does not define you. Your hurt is part of you, and it matters, but it is not who you are at the core of your being. Whatever you have been through, whatever your story is, whatever your addiction may be, whatever hurts and wounds you carry in life, I accept and love you. The love I experience is also inside you.

Love requires that you don't have to be anything, but you.

Chapter Twenty-Nine
The Man of My Dreams

I had always anticipated living on my own without a life partner. It was a foregone conclusion that I would be single. My mother told me from an early age that no man would want me because I was "too big". Over the years I developed some close male friendships which I still value highly, but an intimate male companion was another story.

This was about to change. Out of nowhere, I was swept off my feet. I fell head over heels in love. Nothing could prepare me for what I was about to experience.

I vividly remember the first time I saw him. It was at his parents' home south of Adelaide. I had seen a few pictures of him, but nothing could prepare me for meeting him in the flesh. I was nervous as I pulled up outside his home. My heart raced in anticipation as I stepped out of the car and made my way to the front door. So many questions were in my mind. Would he like me? Would this work out? Would this be the man of my dreams, or a nightmare?

Standing at the front door I hesitated momentarily, gathered myself, and raised my hand to knock, knowing that this could change my life forever. I knocked, stepped back, and waited. The door opened and there he stood! He was even more handsome than the pictures I had seen. He was the most beautiful thing I had ever laid eyes on. I was caught off guard when he excitedly lunged toward me. He was a large fawn greyhound. It was love at first sight.

Admired for their grace and speed, greyhounds are one of the oldest breeds of dogs and have been used in racing since the early 20th century. Retired racing greyhounds need a home. These greys find a second chance at life in loving homes through greyhound adoption programs. Greyhound rescue groups take unwanted or retired racing greyhounds and place them with a foster family to acclimatize them to life after racing. Once the foster process is complete, the greyhound can be adopted by people like myself. Effort is made to match the right dog with the right person.

In my case, it was clear from the beginning that this fawn greyhound and I were a perfect match. His foster parents were sad to see him go but happy he had found someone who loved him. His racing nickname was "Meany". Fee decided it was only fitting that the perfect new name for him was "Dreamy", after all, he was the man of my dreams!

Having lived my adult life on my own, I had a daily routine and kept everything in its place. I was a "neat freak"; I liked things orderly and clean. My life could be divided into two eras: BD (Before Dreamy), and AD (After Dreamy). Life with Dreamy wasn't quite as organized and tidy.

On my way home from adopting Dreamy, he and I stayed with my friend Jean for a few days. He slept with me each night we were there. It was an adjustment sleeping with a large, sprawling, furry body next to me. By the time we left, Dreamy and I were two peas in a pod. But then we got home.

Day One:

- Dreamy explored, sniffed, and rubbed his body against the furnishings in my home.

- Dreamy used the newly installed doggy door to discover the garden.

- Dreamy peed on the rose bushes.
- Dreamy drank from my fishpond.
- Dreamy jumped on my bed.
- Dreamy pissed on an ottoman.

Over the next few days and months, Dreamy kept being Dreamy:

- Dreamy chewed on the door frames.
- Dreamy scratched the walls of the laundry.
- Dreamy ripped 4 beds apart in the laundry.
- Dreamy dug holes in the backyard.
- Dreamy brought mud inside.
- Dreamy vomited on the carpet.
- Dreamy crapped on the carpet.
- Dreamy peed on the rug.
- Dreamy howled when I was away, and the neighbours complained.
- Dreamy pulled on the lead and I hit my face on the pavement. I got a black eye.
- Dreamy took up the whole bed, snored and farted, and I got no sleep.

So much for order and cleanliness. This greyhound was turning my life upside down.

It took time, patience, and understanding for Dreamy and I to work each other out. I was not used to having someone else in my space. At first his size and exuberance frightened me. He would lay on the floor blocking my way and I was scared to step over him.

His lack of respect for my home angered me. When I was away, he chewed his beds. He jumped in my unmade bed when I showered in the morning. One day he managed to pull down the awning over the back door, tearing the canvas. He also ripped out the rubber between the glass sliding doors. He was wrecking my home. Perhaps Meany was a better name for him!

At times I wondered if I could do this, but I knew we were meant to be together. Then I began to understand him. Dreamy and I were alike. Both of us had suffered trauma that we did not deserve. Just as I was born into a family who was indifferent to me, Dreamy was bred to race and then no longer wanted by his owner.

Greyhounds are often kept in oppressive conditions. Some, in warehouse-style kennels in rows of stacked metal cages, forced to spend most of their time alone, confined to a cage for 20-23 hours a day. The cages are barely large enough to stand up or turn around in, and the greyhounds are denied the opportunity to walk or play.

Some racing greys are given drugs to enhance their performance. Many suffer injuries while racing or become ill and are killed rather than receive necessary veterinary care. Dogs are herded into the back of trailers and transported long distances in extreme weather conditions. Sometimes they will die on the road in these crowded, miserable conditions.

I had suffered from anxiety as a result of my trauma, and anxiety is a common behavioural problem in both racing and retired greyhounds. Nervous or fearful behaviour, inappropriate soiling, destructiveness, and excessive barking and howling are all signs of anxiety in a greyhound. Dreamy did all of these. He was also afraid of confined spaces, of loud noises, and flying bugs. Anxiety is a common reason for greyhound adoption failures, with many returned for this reason.

The more I understood Dreamy's history, the more empathy I felt for him. Just like my obesity, greyhound misbehaviour is a complicated matter that is caused by a range of factors, many of which are outside their control. Rather than condemn and be angry with

Dreamy, I sought to understand him, and relate to him with patience and love.

Just as it had been for me, it would take time for Dreamy to overcome his anxiety. I was not going to return him; this would be like giving up on myself. How could I give up on him when others had not given up on me? I was in this for the long haul. We both needed each other.

As weeks and months passed, he improved. Dreamy developed a daily routine, and familiarity gave him a sense of security. I looked forward to his greeting each day that I returned home from work. He was always so happy to see me. I began to notice his sweet and amusing idiosyncrasies.

Dreamy was a cuddler. He was at my side as close as he could possibly get. He followed me to the bathroom and leaned against me as I sat. Sometimes I would sit with him on the couch, and he would lay his head on my lap and fall asleep with a big smile on his face. I often watched him drift off. This is what Dreamy needed most; peaceful rest. It was time for him to relax, heal, and be free.

My home became his too. He roached on my bed. Greyhounds roach when they sleep on their back with all four legs in the air, looking like a dead cockroach. This meant he made himself vulnerable, indicating that he felt perfectly comfortable and safe in his new environment.

Loving and caring for Dreamy, was healing for me. He taught me a lot about unconditional love. Dreamy didn't care if I was underweight or overweight, size 6 or 36, stocky or petite. I gave my heart to him and he gave me his. He liked me to rub his tummy, and as I did, I told him how special he was.

Dreamy taught me about being present in the daily moments of life. He enjoyed laying on the floor, bathing in the sun as it streamed through the window, experiencing the warmth across his body.

Dreamy had a natural capacity to be open to each moment as it unfolded without all the mental commentary and drama we impose on life. He didn't care about yesterday or tomorrow; he was in the moment, enjoying whatever presented itself to him.

Dreamy's presence and love was precious to me when I was hurting emotionally. He knew when I was struggling, and we would cuddle. He would read my cues, watching me. We shared a bond and companionship, which warmed my heart. At night I could hear his breathing beside my bed. The sound relieved the loneliness I sometimes felt in moments of sadness and grief.

He became my new walking partner at the Blue Lake. He loved the outdoors, which was most likely a contrast to his previous life. Dreamy would stop to smell scents from other dogs, flowers and plants, look for rabbits, and was fascinated by distant cattle and sheep feeding in the paddocks surrounding the lake.

Dreamy was a people magnet. Greyhounds were not in abundance where we live, and I had never seen one at the Blue Lake. Their tall, slender, and graceful appearance attracts attention. Everyone at the Blue Lake loved Dreamy. His greyhound way of leaning on people for attention endeared him to those we met. He became familiar with some people and would whine, bark and wag his tail in delight whenever he saw them. At night when we walked together, he would stay close to my side, protecting me from unfamiliar figures in the dark.

I met many people and made new friends because of Dreamy. He was a good icebreaker for the frozen walls we hide behind in public. His eagerness to solicit friendship had a way of opening people's hearts and drawing out their goodness.

Dreamy opened a part of my sole that I had hidden for so long. His innocence, generosity, love, trust, and loyalty were special. He gave so much and asked for so little in return. He didn't judge and was incapable of the flaws I suffered with. He was always there for me, despite how I treated him.

When I adopted Dreamy, I made a promise to care for him. In doing so, I learned more about caring for myself. One of the greatest gifts he gave me was to teach me how to give compassion to myself.

Milan Kundera, author of *The Unbearable Lightness of Being*, wrote, "Dogs are our link to paradise. They don't know evil or jealousy or discontent. To sit with a dog on a hillside on a glorious afternoon is to be back in Eden, where doing nothing was not boring—it was peace."

Dreamy was a constant reminder that I was needed and loved. Time with him connected me with my heart and gave me permission to freely share the love I carried within. Like any relationship, this one had its costs, but rather than get angry or frustrated, I accepted these and balanced them against the joy, love, and companionship he gave me.

As an obese woman, I had been treated abysmally at times. But Dreamy never did this to me.

Will Rogers wrote, "If there are no dogs in Heaven, then when I die, I want to go where they went."

Me too.

Chapter Thirty

The World Is Not Flat

I have been obese since early childhood. For much of my life I have been maligned for my obesity. It came from every front—school, religion, work, social media, and the daily stares of judgment and contempt.

Our society is obsessed with appearance. We have forgotten that we are humans who need love, compassion, dignity, and respect. I have never sought special status, just like everyone else all I wanted was to be treated as a human being.

The Word Health Organization uses the Body Mass Index (BMI) as its main method of determining obesity. BMI is measured by dividing a person's weight in kilograms by the square of their height in metres. If the result is 30 or more, the individual is considered obese. This is the measure most medical professionals use.

The Body Mass Index was developed by a mathematician in the 19th century when the world was still considered flat. He had little medical knowledge at a time when such knowledge was woefully limited.

In my opinion, BMI is one of the most detrimental measures of health ever used on humankind. It is based on the false notion that slender, low weight people are healthier. Factors such as bone structure, muscle mass, and body shape are ignored. Even elite athletes may have a high BMI because they have a lot of muscle mass and fall above the threshold of 30, yet not technically be obese. My body shape is big-boned and broad-shouldered. Most of my weight is carried in the chest cavity. I have a high BMI. I am not a model, yet I am fit, healthy, and not obese. Equating health with slimness is problematic.

The best measure of obesity is the distribution of fat across our body. Excessive fat stored in our abdomen can contribute to health problems such as diabetes and heart disease. At this point in time, very few medical clinics use measures to determine the amount of fat in the abdominal region.

Over the years I have been judged as unmotivated, lazy, indifferent, slow, gluttonous, and unintelligent. Yet, I walk every day, eat healthy, have a higher academic degree, and hold down a job as an accountant.

We are obsessed with body image. Television shows such as The Biggest Loser have contributed to this fixation. Weight loss in a controlled environment where we are shielded from the triggers that cause overeating is not real life. Neither is the support, encouragement, and 24-hour accountability and guidance that the people on these shows receive. Not only is this unrealistic, it is dangerous. Quick weight loss is unsafe and usually results in regaining and adding more weight, as the results of The Biggest Loser demonstrate.

Poor diet and inadequate exercise are not the only factors or even the most important ones that contribute to weight gain and obesity. On the surface, the cause of obesity seems simple: if we consume more calories than we burn as energy through physical activity, then we will gain weight. But this is a simplistic explanation, which shows our ignorance in our understanding of obesity. The risk factors that contribute to obesity are a combination of genetics, socioeconomic factors, metabolic factors, and trauma, among other things.

Coming out of obesity requires a holistic approach to wellbeing which includes physical, mental, emotional, and relational health. There were many factors which contributed to my obesity, including genetics, family history, trauma, stress, sugar addiction, and food sensitivities.

My journey has been about experiencing a love bigger than myself and learning to love myself, my body, and the world around me. I have been healed of my shame and become healthier both inside and out. In the end I learned to have empathy toward my body. It had brought me a long way, despite my unhealthy lifestyle and weight. It has undergone three major surgeries and changes in diet, posture, and weight. My body as it is right now is a symbol of success, not because it's thinner, lighter, and has a better BMI measurement, but because I stopped hating it and learned to accept and love it unconditionally.

One never truly overcomes obesity. Like anorexia, it is a lifelong internal battle. Although I have lost a substantial amount of weight, I still think like an obese person. There are times when I catch myself assuming I am the biggest in the room or covered in rolls of fat. Sometimes I think I'm still markedly different from others. Sometimes I want unhealthy food and think about creating a rich, sweet chocolate cake. But then I remember that I couldn't eat it anyway. Then I remind myself of my journey and clarity returns.

Obesity is not merely a matter of medical science or a physical condition or disease, it's a mental health crisis. Obesity is not the consequence of overeating, it's a symptom of a much deeper problem. We are trapped in obesity not because we lack information about food and health, but because of our self-sabotaging beliefs. Obesity is not a BMI number, it's a cry for help. Shame, alienation, self-hatred, fear of rejection, lack of confidence, and disempowering attitudes are all inner blockages that sabotage the best-made medical plan.

Indian philosopher, Jiddu Krishnamurti, wrote, "It is no measure of health to be well adjusted to a profoundly sick society." Our cultural obsession with thinness is killing us. Every day another teenager develops an eating disorder, harms themselves, or takes their life because they don't have the perfect body.

With the aim of challenging the current attitudes toward obesity, I have contacted organizations which claim to help those struggling with obesity. I was disappointed to find that these agencies were mostly staffed by people who have the same misunderstanding about obesity as I have found elsewhere.

Although I can't change the world, I can do my part. I have studied to become certified as a functional medicine health coach, and I have my own coaching business, working with people who struggle with food issues, body image, and those who want to improve their physical, mental, and emotional wholeness and wellbeing. This book tells my story. I hope it starts a different conversation about the obesity epidemic.

Before and After

8:30 on a Monday night I heard a Messenger notification on my phone. It was a woman with whom I had attended high school. We were both around 17 years of age when we last saw each other, but now she was a middle-aged woman like me. Out of the blue she wanted to meet with me. I had not spoken with her for 37 years.

This seemed odd. I hesitated at first. What did she want? Why did she want to see me after all this time? Despite my conflicted feelings, I agreed.

The next evening, we met up at a local coffee shop. As I stepped inside, I looked for her. I had no idea what she would look like after almost 4 decades since our last contact. Memories of my high school years flooded my mind as I walked through the coffee shop. They were not happy years for me, I could not imagine that this would be a happy conversation.

Then, I heard a voice call my name. She was sitting at a table with her husband. She smiled when I spotted her and jumped up from her seat to greet me. She had seen my pictures on Facebook and expressed how amazed she was by my weight loss. She asked me how I had done it, taking it all in like a sponge.

She told me she had seen a bariatric surgeon. I mentioned that I did not have lap band surgery. She was shocked and said, "What? You did it all on your own? That's amazing!"

She asked me what I felt made the biggest difference in my losing so much weight. My answer was, love. There is nothing that cannot be healed by love. Eventually, we discover that love heals everything, and love is all there is.

Pictures cannot convey the blood, sweat, and tears of my battle with obesity. It seemed much longer than a "journey of a thousand miles". A weight loss photo cannot show the shame I carried, the circumstances that led to my enormous weight gain, or the rejection, abuse, and scorn I suffered throughout my life.

I once thought my journey was about coming out of obesity. But now I know it was always about trusting in divine love, the love we all carry within us. Rumi wrote, "Your task is not to seek for love, but merely to seek and find all the barriers within yourself that you have built against it." Each step in my journey of a thousand miles was chipping away at all the barriers I had built up within myself against love.

I could never have imagined at the beginning of this painful journey that it would end up this way. I would not wish the suffering I have lived with on anyone. But this journey was worth every ounce of pain to discover and know true love within myself.

These days I am grateful for the joy of blending in. Whether it's at the Blue Lake walking Dreamy, on a trip with Fee, or even to the supermarket, no one really notices me. It's nice not being in the spotlight. People go to great measures to be the centre of attention and gain the approval of others.

My greatest wish for you is that you will come to accept, love, and like yourself as you are. You are worthy of that right now, whatever your weight or BMI may be.

Love is your birthright. Love is essentially who you are. The before and after miracle is not what you lost in weight, but what you always had in love.

My journey is proof that love always comes through.

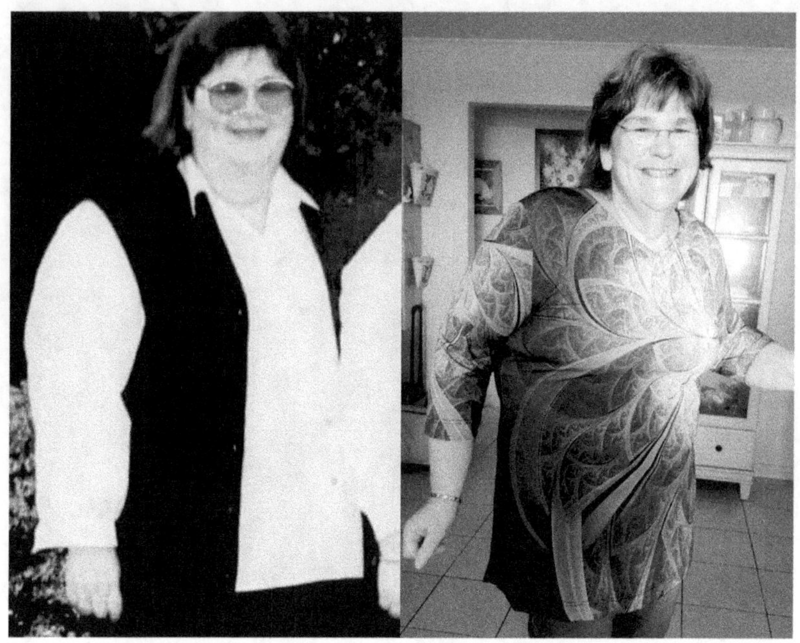

Left: Jenny at her brother's wedding. Credit: Wedding photo owned by Helen Marshall
Right: Jenny after second surgery to remove excess flesh. Credit: Althea Miegel

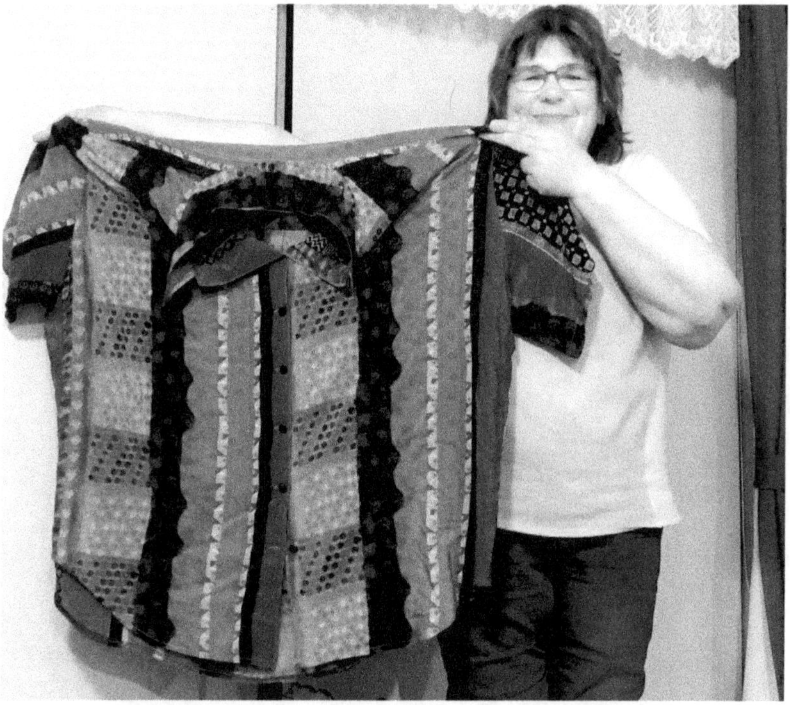

Jenny with her size 32 shirt from the past. Photo Credit: Karren Owen

For more information about Jenny Marshall,
or to contact her for speaking engagements,
please visit *www.JennysThoughts.com*

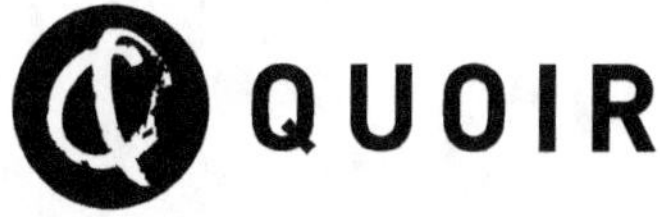
QUOIR

Many voices. One message.

Quoir is a boutique publisher
with a singular message: *Christ is all.*
Venture beyond your boundaries to discover Christ
in ways you never thought possible.

For more information, please visit
www.quoir.com

www.ingramcontent.com/pod-product-compliance
Lightning Source LLC
Chambersburg PA
CBHW052354060726
47592CB00020B/2221